MODERN GYNÆCOLOGY
WITH OBSTETRICS
FOR NURSES

CHAPTER 1

PHYSIOLOGY OF THE FEMALE REPRODUCTIVE SYSTEM

In all mammals, including man, there is a period from birth onwards in which there is steady growth and development of mind and body, while the reproductive system remains immature and dormant. At a time which is relatively constant for the species—and in man this is around the age of ten—a gradual development of the reproductive organs begins, culminating in widespread physical and mental changes, and the stage of sexual maturity is attained in the ensuing years. In the female this maturity is associated with the appearance of regular cyclical changes in the reproductive system, of which the most striking is the rhythmic discharge of blood from the uterus at intervals of about twenty-eight days. This bleeding, or menstruation, continues for about thirty-five years, only interrupted in the healthy by pregnancy. Then the reproductive powers wane, and to the accompaniment once more of physical and mental changes, cessation of menstruation, i.e. the menopause, indicates the close of the fertile period of life.

The physiology involved in this series of changes affects not only the reproductive organs, but the central and autonomic nervous systems and many of the endocrine glands. Since many gynæcological complaints are the result of disturbances of function rather than of organic conditions like infections or new growths, a review of this physiology is important in order to understand symptoms and the reasons for treatment.

Research into the functions of the brain and the endocrine system constantly produces new information on the physiological control of the female sexual rhythm, especially with regard to the role of the pituitary gland and the hypothalamus. There is no doubt that our understanding of these processes will be further expanded by future work.

Throughout childhood while the reproductive activity is in abeyance, a small girl's figure is neuter in type, the breasts are undeveloped and hair is absent from the body. The uterus is small, its body being shorter than the cervix, and the vagina is narrow and its secretion alkaline. The egg cells, or oöcytes, are present in the ovaries, but are dormant. About the age of ten changes become apparent; growth becomes quicker, the pelvis widens, and fat is laid down round the shoulders, breasts and hips. Hair appears on the pubic area and in the axillæ, childish interests and attitudes are gradually abandoned, and when she is twelve or thirteen years old menstruation begins. The endocrine activity that brought about these changes is briefly as follows.

The reproductive cycle is started and controlled by the hypothalamus, and through it by the pituitary gland, which lies in a hollow in the sphenoid bone at the base of the skull. The hypothalamus, as its name implies, lies just below the thalamus, which is a sensory centre, and it is connected below to the stalk of the pituitary gland. The hypothalamus forms the floor of the third ventricle, has a good blood supply because of its endocrine functions, and contains groups of nerve cells which not only make hormones, but also monitor changes in the blood passing through, and regulate metabolic activity (e.g. temperature control and appetite) in accordance with this information.

In connection with long-distance air travel, one often hears about the upset of the daily or Circadian rhythm concerned with sleep, urine output and hormone secretion. This daily rhythm, as well as the monthly female cycle, is controlled by the hypothalamus, acting mainly through the pituitary gland.

The pituitary gland consists of two parts, distinct in structure and function. The posterior part is nerve fibres, the cells of which lie in the hypothalamus, while the anterior part is glandular. Of the many hormones produced by the pituitary, only those concerned with female sex function need be considered here. The hypothalamus stimulates the pituitary to produce oxytocin, which causes contraction of the uterus during the birth of the baby, and helps in lactation by stimulating contraction of the muscles of the milk ducts in the breasts. Synthetic preparations of oxytocin are sometimes used to facilitate delivery, or to control haemorrhage after the baby's birth by contracting the uterine muscle.

THE FEMALE REPRODUCTIVE SYSTEM

The anterior pituitary secretes three hormones, which act on the sex organs, and are therefore known as gonadotrophins. These are:—

(1) Follicle-stimulating hormone, of FSH, is related to the maturing and discharge of an egg-cell or ovum from the ovary into the Fallopian tube, i.e. ovulation.

(2) Luteinizing hormone, or LH, promotes the formation of the corpus luteum and hence the secretion of progesterone.

(3) Prolactin (lactogenic hormone) stimulates the breasts to produce milk after delivery. At other times its manufacture is inhibited by the hypothalamus.

The effect of the pituitary hormones on the ovary is as follows.

The ovary consists of a central portion or medulla, freely

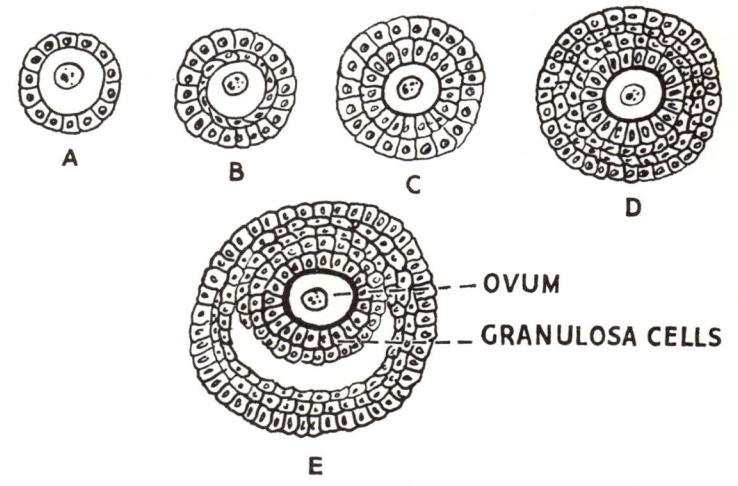

FIG. 4. Stages of development of the Graafian follicle. E shows the follicle distended with fluid, the liquor folliculi, and the ovum surrounded by the granulosa cells.

supplied with blood vessels, and an outer cortex in which lie the egg cells or ova. Under the influence of FSH some of these ova begin to develop and mature. A layer of cells, the follicular epithelium, appears around the ovum, which grows in diameter and is known together with its surrounding cells as a Graafian follicle. Within the follicle a layer of cells called the granulosa cells appears and proliferates, until the follicle is an ovoid structure with the egg cell situated at one side. Spaces appear within the granulosa layer, merge and fill with fluid, until the mature Graafian follicle is a mass of cells distended with fluid, with the egg cell situated inside it attached to one border. During the ovulatory phase stimulated by FSH several such follicles may be seen ripening in the cortex and approaching the surface. They are not all at the same stage of development, and one reaches the surface in advance of the others. The thin wall of the follicle ruptures, and the mature ovum is discharged into the peritoneal cavity and is drawn into the Fallopian tube by the ciliary action and peristalsis of that structure. The other follicles not quite so far advanced in development then begin to degenerate, and are eventually replaced by fibrous tissue.

Ordinarily only one follicle matures and ruptures, but if two ripen simultaneously, two ova enter the Fallopian tube, and if both are fertilized, dissimilar or binovular twins will result. Identical twins result from a single fertilized ovum which has divided at a very early stage. In the event of quintuplets being conceived, at least three follicles must ripen and be fertilized at the same time. A tendency to multiple pregnancies appears to be hereditary.

The ovulatory phase in the ovary is associated with the production in large quantities of one of the ovarian hormones, œstrogen. This hormone is secreted mainly just before and during ovulation, the developing follicle being responsible for the sudden rise in the œstrogen level in the blood. An œstrogen is any substance, natural or artificial, which stimulates proliferative changes in the endometrium. It is certainly produced also before menstruation begins, since the physical changes of puberty are due to its action, **and even after** menstruation has ceased **small quantities are formed.** It is responsible for such secondary sex characteristics as the growth of hair, the development of the labia and clitoris, deposition of fat and development of the breasts. It increases the permeability of the capillaries and causes water retention in the tissues. It stimulates peristalsis in the Fallopian tubes, and is responsible for the acidity of the vaginal secretion in the adult. After menstruation it hastens the regeneration of the denuded epithelium in the uterus.

THE FEMALE REPRODUCTIVE SYSTEM

Many synthetic substances having an action like the normally occurring œstrogen have been made, varying in activity and also in their toxic effects. The clinical uses of these will be considered later.

The ovulatory phase initiated by FSH and characterized by ovulation and a rise in the œstrogen level in the blood occupies about fourteen days, including menstruation; and ovulation takes place about the fourteenth day before the onset of the next period. The second fourteen days, or the other half of the month, are characterized by pregnancy preparations, which are stimulated by pituitary LH.

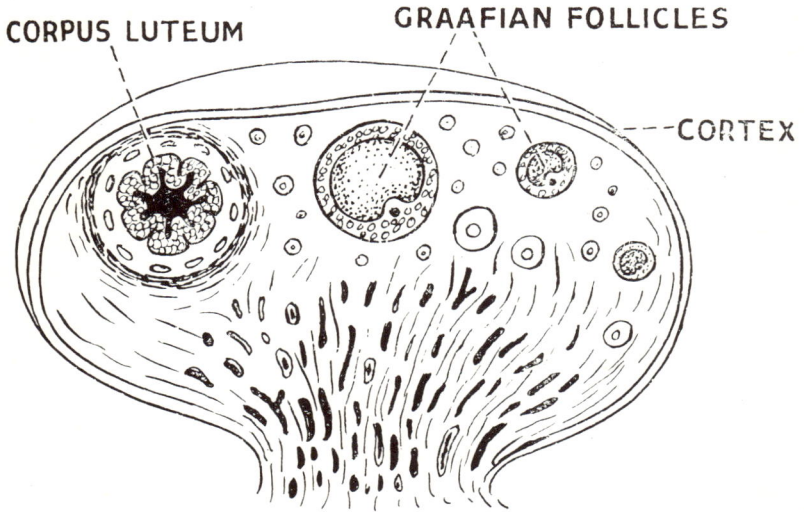

FIG. 5. Diagram of ovary in section.

After the ovum has escaped from the ruptured follicle, the granulosa cells lining the follicle hypertrophy to form a convoluted mass of cells called the corpus luteum, i.e. yellow body. It is a reddish-grey at first, but gradually assumes the yellow colour that its name indicates. The corpus luteum produces the hormone progesterone, whose effects dominate the second half of the reproductive cycle. Briefly, it prepares the endometrium for the reception of a fertilized ovum. The lining of the uterus becomes still thicker and more vascular, and its glands enlarged and tortuous.

The fate of the corpus luteum depends on whether or

not pregnancy has occurred. If it has, the rapidly growing but still minute pregnancy produces a hormone called chorionic gonadotrophin, which is carried by the mother's blood to the pituitary, where it stimulates the production of more LH. Thus the corpus luteum remains and enlarges, and by its progesterone secretion maintains the lining membrane of the uterus to which the new pregnancy is attached, and upon which it depends for its early nutrition and survival. If fertilization fails to occur the ovum passing down the Fallopian tube disintegrates, and the corpus luteum begins to regress, so that progesterone secretion falls away rapidly. The endometrium, which has been built up into a highly developed state by the combined action of the two ovarian hormones, becomes unstable, its surface layers disintegrate, and blood and mucus are discharged from the uterine cavity into the vagina and thence to the exterior. Bleeding will continue for three to five days, becoming less bright and less copious after the first two days, and a quantity varying from 60 to 180 ml. will be lost. Menstruation thus marks the end of an infertile cycle; but even while it is still in progress healing is taking place in the deeper layers of the endometrium, further Graafian follicles are approaching the surface of the ovary, and the whole cycle will be repeated.

Although menstruation indicates the end of a cycle, it is such a well-marked phenomenon that in clinical work the first day of the period is known also as the first day of the cycle. It would be more logical to speak of the date of ovulation as the first day, but in most women this cannot be known with certainty, though it occurs fairly regularly fourteen days before the onset of the next menstrual period. Some women, however, feel abdominal pain (*mittelschmerz*) at the time of ovulation, occasionally severe enough to make them seek medical advice. If the pain is in the right ovary, the patient may be unfortunate enough to be subjected to an operation for supposed appendicitis, which indicates the importance of obtaining a menstrual history from women with abdominal pain. Ovulation, incidentally, occurs from either ovary indiscriminately, and not from each alternately, as is widely believed.

The main events of the reproductive cycle can be summarized in a simple form in this way:—

THE FEMALE REPRODUCTIVE SYSTEM 11

(1) Œstrogen is secreted by the developing follicle; the endometrium begins to regenerate and thicken under the influence of the œstrogen.

(2) The ovum is liberated from the surface of the ovary, and passes into the Fallopian tube.

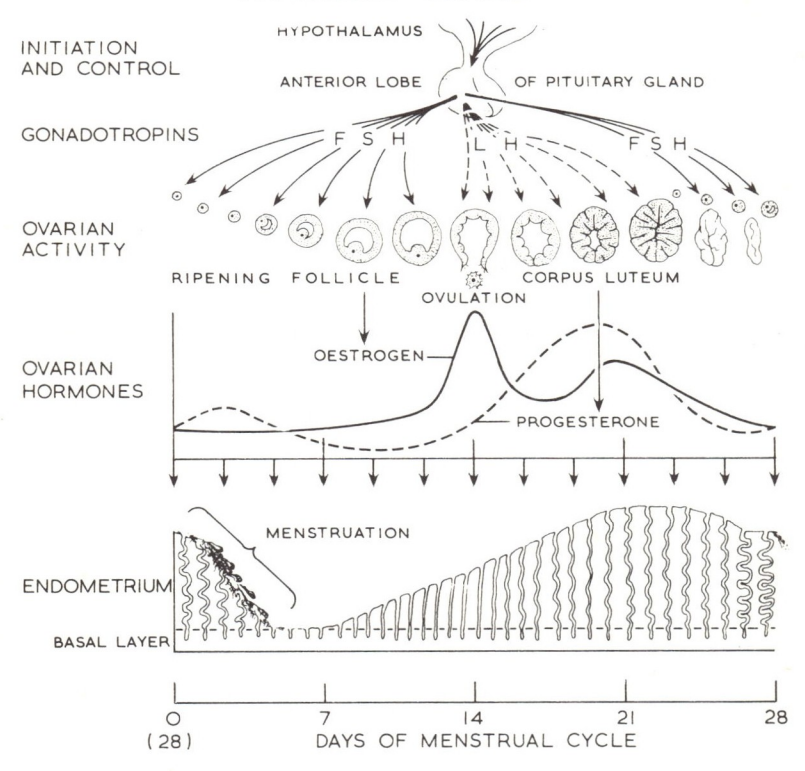

Fig. 6. Diagram to illustrate the female reproductive cycle.

(3) The corpus luteum forms in the ovary and secretes progesterone, which prepares the endometrium for the embedding of a fertilized ovum.

(4) If fertilization does not occur, the corpus luteum degenerates, and the thickened endometrium is cast off fourteen days after ovulation.

(5) This series of events is stimulated by the hypotha-

lamus via the anterior lobe of the pituitary gland, and will occur regularly over a cycle of about twenty-eight days, unless pregnancy occurs.

The endometrium consists of three layers:—

(a) A narrow *basal* layer in contact with the uterine muscle.

(b) An intermediate or *spongy* layer which forms the greater thickness of the ripe endometrium.

(c) A narrow superficial or *compact* layer which acts as a protective covering.

During menstruation the two superficial layers (the spongy and compact) are shed, leaving the basal layer intact, and it is from this narrow layer that the whole endometrium regenerates to form a new cycle.

The uterus thus obeys the endocrine stimulus of the ovary, the ovary that of the pituitary gland, and the pituitary that of the hypothalamus. This structure appears to act as a biological clock, timing many of the body rhythms and through its connections with the nervous and endocrine systems bringing reproductive activity under the influence of many other factors.

PUBERTY AND THE MENARCHE

Puberty is the time of transition between childhood and maturity, but is often loosely used to mean the time of onset of menstruation, for which the proper term is *menarche*. The first period, however, is only one manifestation of changes that have been taking place mentally and physically over the preceding few years. A girl is not sexually mature when she begins to menstruate, because she still has several further years of physical growth and mental development to come. The first few periods are quite often unassociated with any of the common discomforts frequently associated with menstruation, because cycles are anovular—that is, an ovum is not produced.

The management of a girl at this time of life is not simply that of instructing her in the hygiene of menstruation. She is growing rapidly and needs a good protein diet, open-air exercise and enough sleep. This is the time at which the type of school which she is subsequently to attend is being decided and so may be a time of considerable strain and mental worry which should be mitigated as far as possible.

To-day in Britain it would be unusual for a girl to arrive at the *menarche* ignorant of the elementary facts of physiology involved; and it would be most undesirable that she should. She needs instruction in simple hygiene; she must be encouraged not to associate invalidism with this natural function, but must be told that exercise, normal life and a healthy physical and mental outlook are essential. External protection is essential during the first few periods, but later external pads or intravaginal tampons may be used according to personal taste and convenience. Some discussion of the use of tampons during menstruation will be found on page 153.

The onset of puberty is the beginning of the difficult phase of adolescence, and wise and careful handling now may avert grief to the girl and her parents also. She begins to want to lead a life of her own, is resentful of questions about her activities, and may cause much distress to a mother who prided herself that her daughter had no secrets from her. The girl wants to make her own experiments with friends and clothes, and though these may seem deplorable to her parents, they should be careful how their criticism is expressed, since gulfs may be opened up now which will be difficult to bridge later on. Beneath the adolescent's veneer of self-confidence she is extremely vulnerable.

Home should be everything in the daughter's life; now it is a base from which she makes sallies into the outside world, and to which she can retreat for a time if her experiments lead to her being hurt. If now she thinks of her home as a safe and happy harbour, not as a threat to her individuality and privacy, the period of adolescence will be an easy one. The constant cry of girls at this age is: " My mother thinks I am still a child "; while mothers say: " My daughter thinks she is grown up." The main adjustment will have to be made by the mother, since wisdom cannot be expected in the girl, who anyway will find that time is on her side and will prove her right.

The adolescent in modern society occupies an important and invidious position. Her earning power is often considerable, and as she has few responsibilities much pressure is exerted on her through all advertising media to spend

14 MODERN GYNÆCOLOGY FOR NURSES

her money. She is hurried, not unwillingly, into an adult world with which she is often unable to cope without support. The rising incidence of venereal disease and of illegitimate births among teenagers suggest that we have somehow failed to give this support, or to offer these girls a moral standard that they can accept.

FERTILIZATION AND PREGNANCY

Every month when the mature ovum is released from the ovary, the uterus is prepared for pregnancy, and the endometrium under the influence of the ovarian hormone is thickened and vascular. When fertilization of the ovum takes place, it occurs in the Fallopian tube by a single

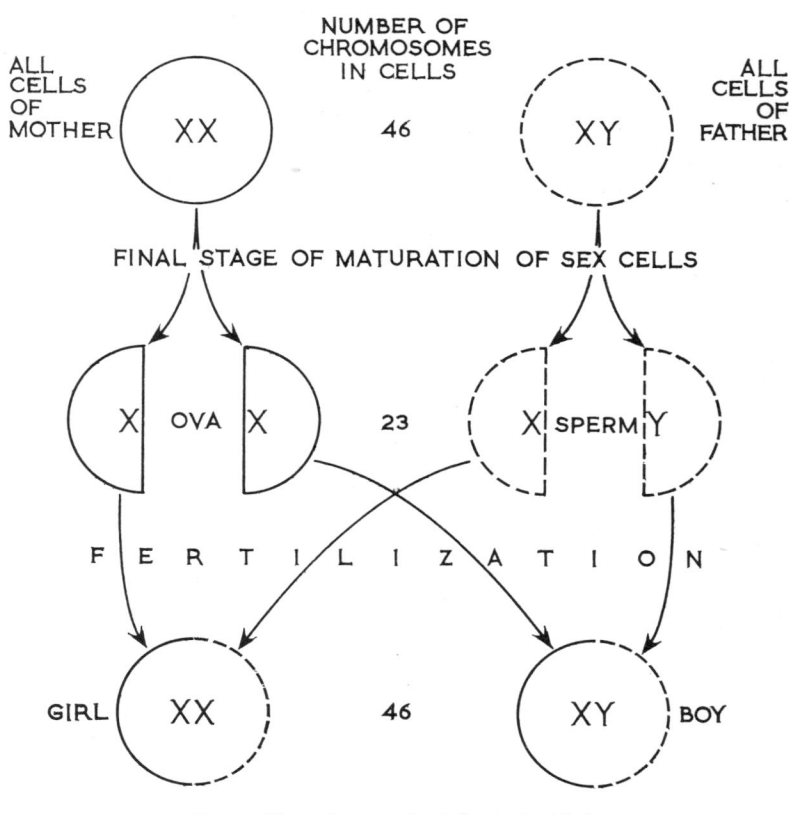

Fig. 7. How the sex of a baby is decided.

THE FEMALE REPRODUCTIVE SYSTEM

spermatozoon after ovulation, and the sex of the baby is determined at its conception in the following way.

Inherited characteristics are handed on to a baby from its parents by means of the *genes*, carried on the *chromosomes* which are part of every cell nucleus. In the human there are normally twenty three pairs of chromosomes. Of these, twenty two pairs (the *autosomes*) transmit such characteristics as eye and hair colour and height; the other pair are the sex chromosomes, which determine whether the owner is male or female. In women the pair are identical, and because of their shape are called X chromosomes. In men the pair are dissimilar, and (again because of their shape) are called XY.

During the final stage of maturation of the ova or spermatozoa, there is a reduction by half of the number of chromosomes, so that these special reproductive cells are unique in the body in containing only twenty three chromosomes, one of which is a sex one. In the ovum this is always an X chromosome, but in the spermatozoon there is an even chance that it is X or Y. The fertilized ovum will therefore have its full complement of twenty three pairs, half from each parent. Of the sex pair, it always has an X chromosome from its mother, but the second one may be X or Y, depending on which sort the spermatozoon possessed. The fertilized ovum may therefore have an XX pair, and will be a girl, or an XY pair, and be a boy.

Abnormal inheritance of sex chromosomes is not always incompatible with life, and extra X or Y chromosomes may be present. If only an extra X chromosome is present the patient is short, with webbing of the neck, female in appearance, but sterile because the ovaries are rudimentary. This condition is called Turner's syndrome. It is possible to determine the sex chromosomes of an individual by staining and examining cells from the mucous membrane inside the cheek, or from the skin. This examination is occasionally required if a baby's external genitalia are unusual, in order to decide if its cell sex is male or female.

Peristalsis and the action of the ciliated lining of the tube conveys the fertilized ovum onwards into the uterus, where it is to live and grow during the forty weeks of pregnancy. The story of the baby's development in the uterus until the time of birth will be found in Chapter 12.

CLIMACTERIC AND THE MENOPAUSE

The normal menopause occurs in one of three ways.

(1) Previously regular periods may cease abruptly and never recur.

(2) The periods may occur at longer intervals, but with a normal amount of bleeding, or a reduced loss.

(3) The periods remain regular, but the amount of loss gradually diminishes until it ceases altogether.

Other variations of the menstrual cycle occurring at the menopause must be considered as abnormal. For instance:

(1) A time during which menstruation occurs at shorter intervals than usual (epimenorrhœa) may precede the menopause.

(2) Heavy loss is sometimes experienced—menopausal menorrhagia.

(3) Irregular bleeding may occur, and although this does not mean that disease is present, such an occurrence raises a point that is of vital importance to nurses whose advice is often asked by anxious women. **If it were possible to teach nurses only one fact in gynæcology, it should undoubtedly be that women complaining of irregular vaginal bleeding, especially at the menopause, should be examined by a specialist in gynæcology, with a view to excluding the presence of malignant disease. If this is stressed more than once in this book, it is because nurses are often in a position to save life by offering the correct advice.**

The climacteric usually starts a year or two before the menopause occurs and lasts for two or three years after it has finished. A woman of placid disposition will often fail to experience any abnormal associated symptoms. Frequently there is a change in the body contours; weight may be lost, or additional fat may be deposited, especially over the shoulders and hips, with loss of tone in the abdominal muscles, but otherwise there may be no complaints. Any of the following symptoms may, however, arise:—

(1) Psychological upsets of various kinds, which result from difficulty in adjustment to her new psycho-sexual environment. She may complain of depression, uncontrollable tearfulness, headache, lassitude and insomnia.

THE FEMALE REPRODUCTIVE SYSTEM

In some cases the depression may be severe enough to be called a psychotic illness. A woman who was psychologically unstable before the climacteric is liable to become worse at this time, and is not helped by popular literature and the lay press suggesting that she is at a critical era in her life.

(2) Vaso-motor symptoms—so-called " hot flushes." These usually start as waves of heat associated with redness of the skin of the face and neck, and they may sweep as a feeling of great heat and oppression over the whole body. Sweating sometimes occurs. In a severe instance, these hot flushes are almost continuous and occur twenty or thirty times a day. If mild, they may last for a few minutes only once or twice a day, or even less frequently, and will eventually be unnoticed. They may go on for months or even years, starting before and continuing after the menopause. They are extremely embarrassing and distressing to the patient, and may cause lack of sleep at night.

(3) An increase of weight is common and is often associated with arthritis, usually in the knee joints, perhaps because increasing weight places an added strain on joints that have been overburdened for many years.

(4) Relaxation of ligaments adversely affects joints and may cause some dropping of the shoulder girdle, scoliosis of the spine, or genital prolapse.

(5) Gastro-intestinal upsets, such as constipation, flatulence or dyspepsia.

(6) Vague neurological symptoms, such as tingling and numbness in the arms and legs, may occur.

With the cessation of ovarian function, the genital tract undergoes a steady and progressive atrophy. The labia minora shrink and become flattened, the vagina becomes progressively narrowed; the epithelium lining the vagina and vulva is thinned and the vulva shrinks, while the uterus and cervix become smaller. Microscopical examination of the ovary shows that all follicle formation has ceased and that it consists entirely of stroma and fibrous tissue. It must not be thought, however, that these changes occur suddenly. It often takes many years for the post-menopausal state to be reached. During this time, the ovary does provide some internal secretions which are of great value to the woman in leading her slowly into the post-menopausal state without an undue or sudden necessity for physiological and psychological adjustment.

THE MANAGEMENT OF THE MENOPAUSE AND CLIMACTERIC

(1) The Menopause. A careful history of the character of the bleeding must be taken, since this is a time at which women are liable to develop cancer of the cervix or body of the uterus. Any irregularity is thoroughly investigated by a gynæcologist. If he is in the slightest doubt as to whether the condition is normal, the patient must be admitted to hospital for further investigation such as biopsy of the cervix, and curettage, or scraping, of the uterine cavity. Only by such precautions will cancer of the uterus be diagnosed in an early and treatable condition.

Some patients with heavy loss towards the menopause will be found on curettage to be suffering from metropathia hæmorrhagica described on p. 99, and of these some will need removal of the uterus. This radical operation is particularly justified when the blood loss is excessive. Most patients, however, who suffer from this condition may subsequently be treated by conservative means, if carefully observed and examined at regular intervals.

(2) The Climacteric. The management is not always easy as the vast mass of proprietary medicines available to the medical and lay public will testify.

(a) Since this is a period of difficult readjustment, the first approach should be simple psychotherapeutic reassurance and explanation of the true situation to the patient in terms which she will understand. Often the middle forties are a time of stress and anxiety apart from the physical changes involved in the climacteric. Perhaps the children are now growing up, leaving home and marrying, and a woman who has been the centre of a busy, happy home, may find that she and her husband are suddenly alone in a home that seems rather big for them. The husband still has his work, but she may find time hanging heavily, and has plenty of opportunity to worry over herself and her husband's attitude to her changing state. Perhaps family cares have left her little time for outside pursuits,

THE FEMALE REPRODUCTIVE SYSTEM

and now that she has the time she has no inclination, or no interests, to fill the gap.

Women who are unmarried now begin to realize that they are unlikely to advance any further in their work, and that if they became unemployed it might be difficult to obtain another post. They may worry over how they are to support themselves in their old age, how to combat loneliness, or what to do about ailing parents. The physician views their problems broadly, and never considers his patient merely as a case of failing reproductive powers.

(*b*) Simple hygienic readjustment, such as attention to the bowels, diet and exercise, will usually pay a handsome dividend.

(*c*) In the more severely disturbed and nervous patient, small doses of a sedative, such as phenobarbitone, are of the greatest help.

(*d*) For all patients in whom hot flushes are a distressing symptom, small doses of an œstrogen are most helpful. In connection with the use of such a drug a very important fact must be noticed. If a woman is given large doses for a long time and then the drug is stopped, bleeding will take place from the uterus (œstrogen withdrawal bleeding). If this happens after the periods have ceased for some time the suspicion of malignancy is of course aroused, and in order to dispel it diagnostic curettage may have to be performed. This gives rise to anxiety in the patient.

CHAPTER 2

EXAMINATION OF THE PATIENT

POSITIONS USED DURING EXAMINATION AND OPERATION

The position in which a patient is most comfortable during an examination is usually that from which the surgeon can gain the information he needs, and great care should be taken in arranging her. The positions most used in gynæcological examinations and operations are as follows:

(1) **Dorsal.** The patient lies on her back with not more than two pillows under her head. The trunk should

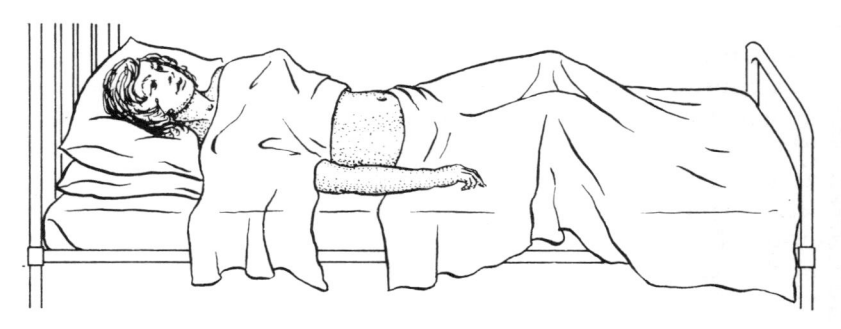

Fig. 8. Dorsal position.

be straight, and the arms by the sides. Examination of the chest, breasts and abdomen is done in this position. The hips may be flexed and abducted to allow vaginal examination to be performed.

(2) **Left Lateral.** The patient is turned on her left side, her knees flexed and her buttocks brought to the edge of the bed or couch. The trunk is somewhat flexed and a pillow drawn under the head. It is important that she is comfortable and relaxed, and the coverings should be arranged to prevent undue exposure while allowing easy access. This attitude is suitable for rectal and vaginal examination.

EXAMINATION OF THE PATIENT 21

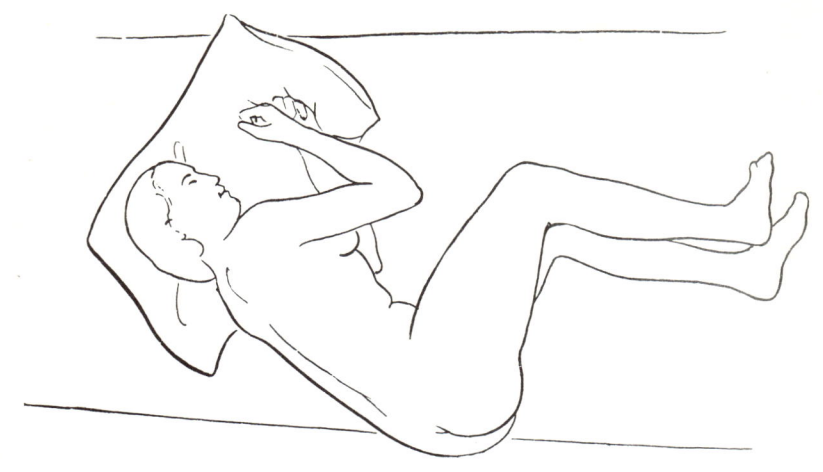

FIG. 9. Left lateral position. In this and subsequent figures coverings have been omitted for the sake of clearness.

(3) **Sims' Position.** If the left lateral position is modified as follows, a better view of the vulva is obtained, and when a speculum has been inserted, the vagina is more easily inspected. The right knee is further flexed, until it lies on the bed above the left one. The left arm is drawn behind the patient so that she lies on her chest. The nurse must see that both arms are comfortable.

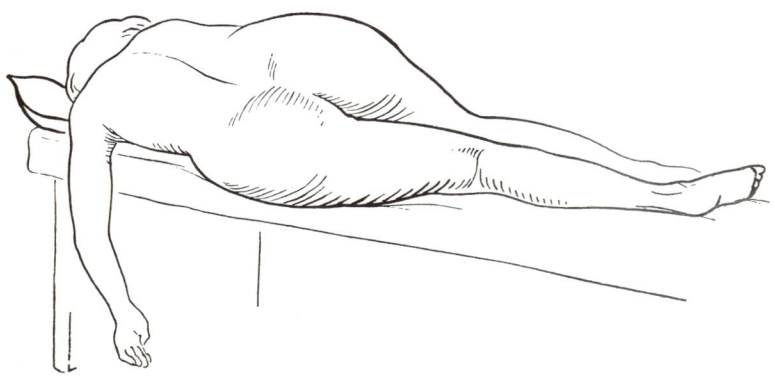

FIG. 10. Sims' position.

(4) **Lithotomy.** This word means "stone cutting," and is a reminder of the days when stone in the bladder was approached from the perineum. The patient lies on

her back, with thighs fully flexed and abducted, and knees flexed. It is most used in the theatre for operations on the vagina and perineum. The end of the table is dropped, the buttocks brought to the edge, the legs supported by fastening the feet to the lithotomy poles by webbing straps round the ankles and insteps. Forceps delivery may be performed in this position, and a variety of general surgical operations on the anus and rectum. It is frequently employed in out-patient clinics in the investigation and treatment of vaginal discharge. A special table may be used with metal troughs for leg support.

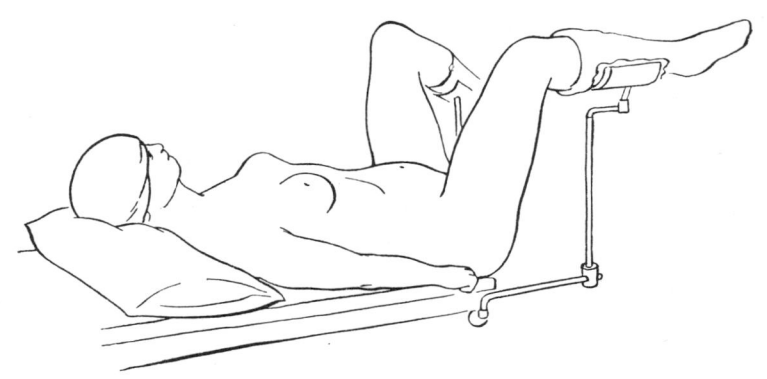

FIG. 11. Lithotomy position.

(5) **Trendelenburg.** The Trendelenburg position is becoming less popular because advances in anæsthesia and surgical technique make it unnecessary. The essence of this position, which is much used in the theatre, is that the head end of the table is lowered, allowing the abdominal organs to move up towards the diaphragm. It is used for the abdominal approach to the pelvic organs, which are better exposed than in the horizontal position. It is obvious that the patient needs to be secured in this position, and there are four ways in which this may be done:—

(1) The most modern and the safest method is the use of Langton Hewer's non-slip corrugated mattress. This enables the patient to be tilted to 45 degrees without any other support except the adhesion of the skin (which must be dry) of the back, buttocks and thighs to the mattress. Supporting cushions of foam rubber covered with the

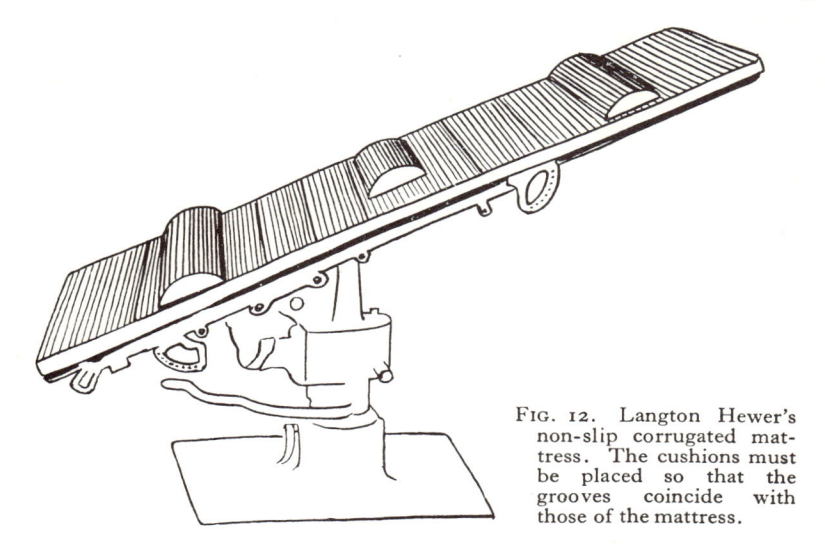

EXAMINATION OF THE PATIENT

Fig. 12. Langton Hewer's non-slip corrugated mattress. The cushions must be placed so that the grooves coincide with those of the mattress.

same corrugated surface are placed as an additional support under the tendines Achillis, the loin and the neck.

The legs are lightly secured against lateral displacement and kept straight. This has the great advantage of unimpeded venous return, and may play a big part in preventing post-operative phlebothrombosis. The arms may be placed across the chest or kept beside the patient's trunk by special malleable metal supports well padded, or rubber straps, so that no prolonged pressure during the operation can damage the nerves or impede the crculation.

If the arm is needed for intravenous infusion, and is exposed by abduction on a wooden splint placed under the patient, it is vital that the abduction must never for a moment exceed 80 degrees, and preferably it should be much less. Brachial palsy can easily result from excessive abduction, and a case of liability for damages may ensue.

(2) Pelvic crest supports can be used to prevent displacement, but are not very satisfactory for the fat patient.

(3) The table end may be dropped to 90 degrees, the knees flexed and the ankles strapped. Pressure on the calves is unavoidable, and this method is not recommended.

(4) Shoulder supports, with or without knee flexion, will maintain the position. Brachial palsy is again a risk if much weight is put on the rests.

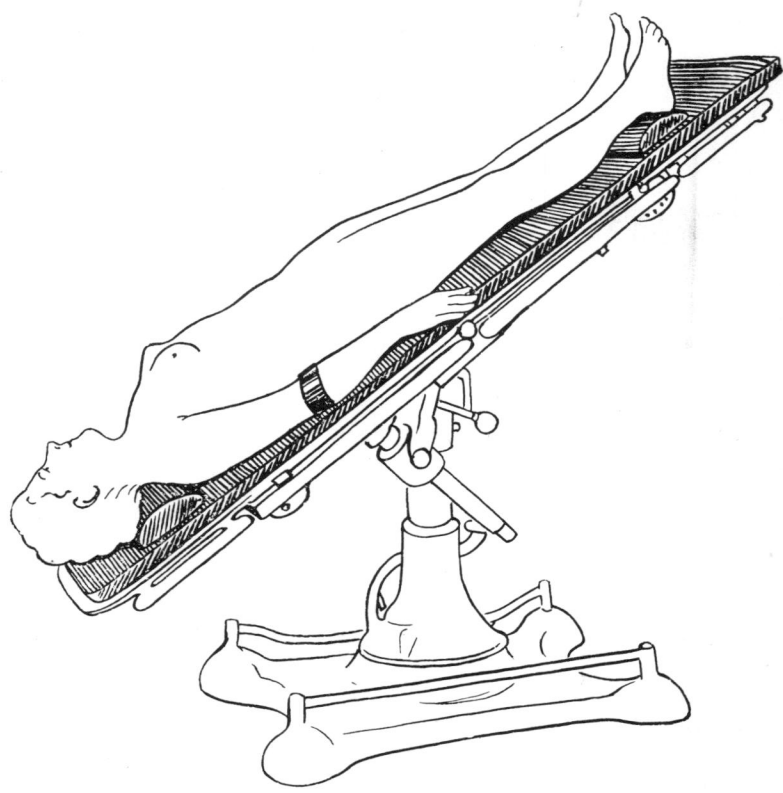

FIG. 13. Patient in Trendelenburg position. The nurse must see that the mattress is hooked to the end of the table before lowering the head.

EXAMINATION OF THE GYNÆCOLOGICAL PATIENT

Such an examination is not confined to the pelvic organs: the patient has to be considered as a whole, or the gynæcologist may find himself treating some local symptoms and missing the primary disease, such as carcinoma of the breast or intestinal tract with ovarian metastases, that is causing them.

The equipment that will be needed and used for a vaginal examination will vary according to whether it is conducted in a ward, an out-patient clinic or at home; on the nature of the information sought, and on the presence or otherwise of a discharge. In some cases where full

EXAMINATION OF THE PATIENT

relaxation is essential, an anæsthetic is given and the examination is conducted in the theatre. If the patient is a young girl, rectal examination is made instead of a vaginal one.

When preparing the trolley given below, it should be remembered that the vagina is not sterile, and full aseptic technique is unnecessary except in the later stages of pregnancy, in the puerperium, or patients suffering from abortion. All non-disposable equipment must be sterilized after use, and it should be borne in mind that in a clinic, where a proportion of patients have a vaginal infection, it is possible to spread such infections unless scrupulous hygiene is observed.

It is desirable for a vaginal examination that the rectum should be empty, and the bladder should be emptied shortly beforehand unless there is a urethral discharge to be examined or the patient complains of prolapse. The urine should always be tested. If a discharge is present a clean pad should be given, and a soiled one saved for inspection. A shawl or blanket is necessary to cover the patient during examination, and if it is taking place on a couch a towel, which may well be a disposable paper one, is provided.

Trolley. Bowl of lotion, such as cetrimide.
  Bowl of swabs.
  Instrument tray with: Specula—Cusco's, Sims',
    Ferguson's
    Spongeholding forceps
    Volsellum forceps
    Proctoscope
  Lamp
  Disposable gloves, powder and lubricant
  Rectal tray
  Receivers for soiled dressing and used instruments.
If a bacteriological examination is to be made, a tray should be added with the following:—
  Rack with throat swabs
  Platinum loop
  Spirit lamp and matches
  Slides and coverslips
  Normal saline and dropper
  Stuart's transport medium and charcoal swabs (for gonorrhœa).

A microscope should be available, so that wet films of any discharge can be examined immediately. Vaginal and cervical smears are usually taken for cytological examination, so the tray should also include Ayre spatulæ, and containers filled with ether-alcohol fixing solution for the slides.

Procedure. The nightgown is removed and the patient lies on her back with a pillow under the head, covered with a blanket, and with the bedclothes turned down to the level of the pubis. The doctor will look at the mucosa of eyes and palate to see if obvious anæmia is present, and then feel the thyroid gland, disorders of which are a cause of menstrual upsets.

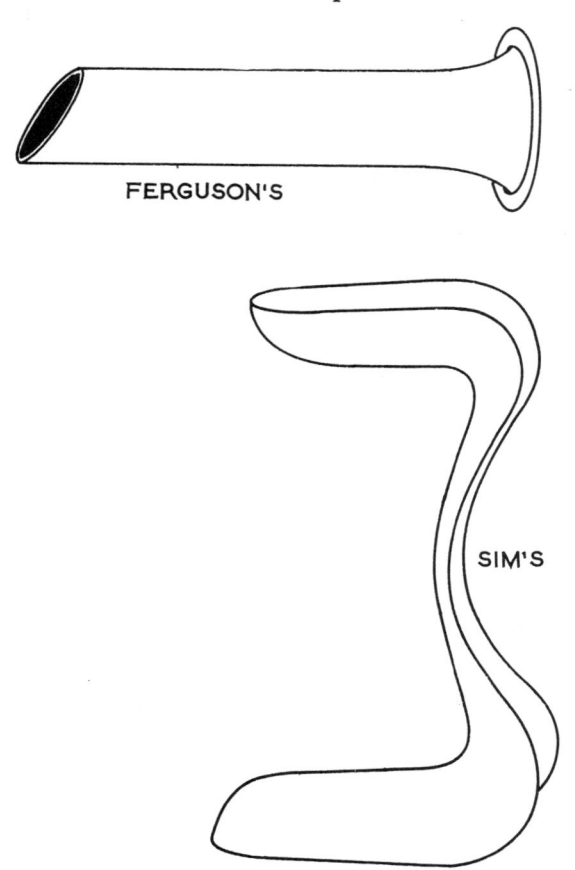

FIG. 14. Vaginal specula.

EXAMINATION OF THE PATIENT

The nurse uncovers the chest, and he examines the breasts for signs of activity that might indicate pregnancy, and if it is indicated he examines the heart and lungs. The chest is covered, and he makes a careful examination of the abdomen. Many pelvic tumours can be felt from the abdomen, including the pregnant uterus after the first twelve weeks. Secondary deposits from malignant pelvic tumours may be palpable.

Vaginal examination follows next, and the nurse places the patient in the selected position, reassuring her that no pain will be felt, while the doctor puts on his gloves. After inspection he will swab the vulva, if necessary, and make first a digital and then a speculum examination. A plain metal speculum and a separate light is commonly used. A Coldite speculum with an illuminated lower blade gives a better view, and best of all is provided by a Fibrelight cable. When it is finished the nurse sees that her patient is dry, and supplied, if necessary, with a clean pad. If a cervical swab or smear has been taken, she must see that it is labelled and sent to the laboratory without delay.

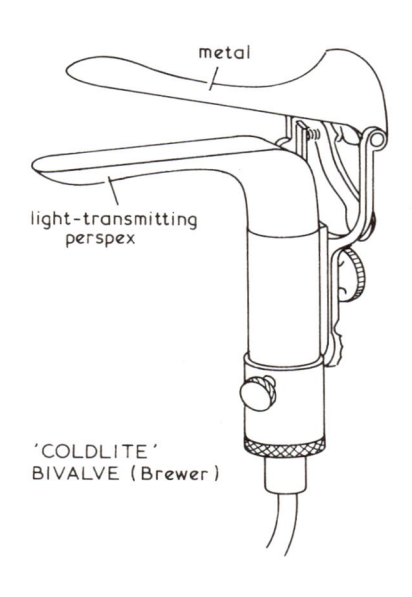

Fig 15. A bivalve Coldlite speculum.

CHAPTER 3

PRE-OPERATIVE TREATMENT

Women's out-patient clinics treat a great variety of complaints, but gynæcological wards contain mostly women having surgical operations for new growths, chronic infections or displacements of the pelvic organs, patients for investigations under anæsthetic, and women threatened with abortion or its consequences who need nursing with aseptic technique. Consideration of the methods used in preparing patients for gynæcological operations must therefore be of importance to the nurse, who will find that general questions of preparation are as vital as in all branches of surgery, while local preparation is more extensive than in many other fields. In this chapter and the next many procedures are described some of which are used progressively less often in modern centres, but all of which a nurse may need to know in some circumstances. Gynæcological nursing must not be thought of as predominantly procedure-centred because such a number of techniques are described. They are merely tools which may be required in the care of a particular woman for whose physical, mental and social needs they may be used.

The consent of the patient to operation is important to all surgeons, but is especially so to the gynæcologist. Once an operation has been decided upon its scope should be carefully explained to her in terms that she can understand. Her written consent is obtained on a form, and that of the husband too is frequently requested, especially if the operation may involve sterilization. If she is a minor, a parent or guardian should preferably sign the form. The legal age of majority was lowered in 1968 from twenty one to eighteen, and if the patient is younger than this the written consent of a parent or guardian to the operation must normally be obtained. In certain circumstances, however, the Department of Health and Social Security allows young people of sixteen to sign their own consent forms, and it is especially in the gynæcological ward that this may arise, principally in connection with pregnancy or abortion in unmarried girls who do not want their parents to know of their state. The principal concern of the surgeon will be the welfare of his patient not only in the present circumstances, but in the future; it is desirable that the parents be as fully consulted as possible about treatment affecting all girls below the age of twenty one. If the patient has cancer, the surgeon exercises his judgement in deciding whether to tell her or no, but in any case the closest relative should be informed of the true nature of the condition.

The gynæcological patient will naturally be anxious as to the exact nature of any operation which it is proposed to perform upon her. For example, a young woman will want to know what effect removal of the womb will have on her as a wife, apart from the obvious loss of reproductive capacity. Many women regard hysterectomy as synonymous with a surgical menopause, and the nurse in charge of such a patient should reassure her that hysterectomy without removal of the ovaries does not affect the sexual life except in so far as it produces permanent cessation of menstruation and reproductive function. She will not suffer from hot flushes, a tendency to obesity, or the psychological symptoms traditionally ascribed to the change of life.

Similarly, a patient still in the reproductive period who undergoes an operation for prolapse will want to know what effect it will have on future childbearing. Nurses should realize that conservative operations performed for prolapse without removal of the womb do not affect marital relations or preclude the possibility of conception. Myomectomy, or removal of a fibroid from the uterus, is another operation which is not sterilizing. Neither do operations such as removal of one tube or ovary prevent further conception, so long as one healthy tube and ovary and the uterus are conserved, and this applies even when, for example, the right tube and the left ovary have been removed.

In general, gynæcological patients undergoing any but minor surgery should be admitted at least forty-eight hours before operation, and the time necessary for adequate investigation and preparation may well be longer. Like all surgical patients, they respond well to a period in which they may accustom themselves to ward routine, and to the doctors and nurses who are to attend them.

During these days a record of the temperature, pulse and respiration is kept, and a final examination is made, especially of the heart and lungs, in view of the forthcoming anæsthetic. The hæmoglobin is estimated, and if operation is a major one the blood group, including the Rhesus typing, is ascertained. When cancer of the cervix is present an intravenous pyelogram is performed and the blood urea estimated in order to exclude the possibility that the ureters are involved in the growth.

If anæmia is severe, it will be corrected by blood transfusion. It is vital in women of child-bearing age that the donor's blood is of the correct Rhesus group, since to give a Rhesus negative patient Rhesus positive blood might have a disastrous effect on subsequent pregnancies and transfusions. If she is suffering heavy menstrual losses, the hæmoglobin must be raised to a satisfactory level by transfusion, and operation soon undertaken before the ground gained is lost once more. It used to be considered not advisable to operate on patients whilst they are menstruating, but this applies today only to operations such as repair or myomectomy.

The patient should be encouraged to move about the ward as much as possible, unless bed rest is prescribed, as for patients with severe prolapse. Exercise has a beneficial effect on the circulation and respiration, and complete inactivity before operation may have serious consequences post-operatively.

The condition of the chest may need treatment, especially if there is any chronic bronchitis, and the physiotherapist is most qualified to help her cough up any secretions. All patients should be taught breathing exercises with a view to obtaining good ventilation of the lungs after operation, and it is desirable to discourage smoking.

In all gynæcological patients, investigation of kidney and bladder function is important. A fluid balance chart must be kept and a note made of the frequency of micturition. If frequent, painful micturition indicates a urinary infection, a mid-stream or clean specimen of urine is sent for culture, and treatment specific to the infecting organism is given. A mixture of potassium citrate and hyoscyamus is valuable before operation, because the hyoscyamus reduces bladder spasm, and the potassium citrate renders the urine

PRE-OPERATIVE TREATMENT

alkaline, and so less liable to infection by *Escherichia coli*, which is the commonest invader of the urinary tract. The patient is encouraged to drink fluids freely before operation in order to wash the bladder out from above, and so minimize the risk of infection.

It is essential that the bladder is quite empty in a patient undergoing gynæcological surgery. The natural function cannot be relied on since many patients cannot completely empty the bladder, and urine may accumulate while the patient is awaiting operation after being prepared. Some surgeons prefer to catheterize the patient in the theatre after the induction of anæsthesia. Otherwise, a catheter may be passed in the ward, spigotted and strapped to the thigh. It should be a soft plastic one, size 7 or 8 for an adult. A smaller one is not more comfortable, and makes it difficult to tell when the bladder is completely empty. It is easy to injure a full bladder while operating in the pelvis and such an injury may seriously prejudice the operation, and will certainly require post-operative bladder drainage. The nurse who is entrusted with pre-operative catheterization must realize how great is her responsibility. She must also see that no patient goes to the theatre without the urine having been tested for albumin and sugar. An operation on an undiagnosed diabetic might end in disaster.

A high fluid intake is desirable not only with regard to the urinary function, but also to help prevent shock after operation. Glucose should be given with the same end in view. The diet should be good, especially with regard to protein, but should not be bulky, and in the case of patients having vaginal operations should be low in residue for the day before going to the theatre. Vitamin C helps healing, and is given as ascorbic acid 50–100 mgm. three times a day.

It is important that the sigmoid colon and rectum are empty, and in vaginal operations it is imperative. Purgatives that entail dehydration are not used, but a simple aperient like cascara is given thirty-six hours beforehand, so that only rarely need an enema be given the night before operation. Distension with flatus is especially to be avoided, and is another reason why mild exercise before operation is beneficial.

The preparation of the skin depends on the surgeon's

wishes, but in all patients undergoing abdominal operation the abdomen and pubic area are shaved, and in those having vaginal operations the vulva must also be shaved. This must be done thoroughly and carefully. With the patient lying on her back with her chest covered with a blanket, the abdomen and pubic area is shave first. The patient is then asked to flex and abduct her thighs, and the nurse takes a large swab in her left hand and covers the vulva except for the left labium majus. This swab is used to keep the skin taut while the left side is shaved, and the right is then similarly treated. The patient is finally turned into the left lateral position, and any hair in the anal region removed. The procedure is not pleasant, and the nurse should take pains to acquire a deft technique.

After the shave, the patient has a bath and the operation area must be thoroughly washed with soap; special attention is paid to the umbilicus. Most surgeons require no further preparation of the skin until the patient is in the theatre, but some expect the skin of the abdomen to be cleaned with some antiseptic lotion, before a sterile towel is bandaged into position over it on the morning of operation.

If a vaginal operation is to be performed, some local preparation is often given, but there is an increasing tendency to omit ward preparation. Vaginal douches were at one time generally used, and are still required in some cases. Painting the vagina is sometimes ordered and the insertion of packs or medicated pessaries may be necessary. All three procedures are described here.

> *Vaginal douche.* The solutions used may be flavine 1 in 1,000; normal saline, or lactic acid 1%. The solution is prepared at a temperature of 40°C (105°F.)
>
> The nurse prepares the following equipment:—
> Douche can, tubing, clip and douche nozzle or catheter size 12.
> Lotion thermometer
> Jug with 1,000 ml. of selected lotion
> Cetrimide for vulval swabbing
> Packet of large swabs
> Waterproof and clinical sheet

PRE-OPERATIVE TREATMENT

Warm douche pan and cover
Blanket or bed jacket

Curtains are drawn round the bed, and if it is the first time of giving the treatment, the nurse assures her patient that it is not uncomfortable. She turns the bedclothes down on to the thighs, and sees that her patient is covered with a blanket or shawl. The pillows are adjusted so that when the mackintosh and towel and douche pan are slipped beneath the buttocks the patient is flat, with the head and shoulders comfortably supported.

The nurse then washes and dries her hands, pours the lotion into the can, allows some to run through the nozzle to expel all air, and tightens the clip. The temperature is checked, and the can adjusted at a height of not more than a foot above the vagina; it may be left on the trolley, or if this is a low one the bowl may be inverted and the can placed on it. It is wrong to think that the solution must be run in under pressure. Too much force may mean that the fluid enters the uterus, which is dangerous, since it may force air into the uterus, and thence into the circulation, causing air embolus, or force lotion to enter the tubes, carrying infected material from the vagina and causing salpingitis. This is an especial risk if the cervix is open, e.g. in an incomplete abortion, or following pregnancy.

The labia minora are parted with the first two fingers of the left hand, and the vaginal orifice swabbed clean with warm lotion. The douche nozzle is taken in the right hand, inspected to see that it is not cracked, and introduced over the perineum into the vagina. The direction of the vagina is backwards towards the sacral promontory, and the nozzle is passed in this direction until it is in the posterior fornix, the clip loosened and the solution allowed to flow in.

When it has run through, the nozzle is removed and returned to the can. Care should be taken not to crack it against the side; these nozzles are fragile, and some surgeons prefer the use of a rubber catheter for this reason. The patient is now assisted to sit up on the douche pan and asked to cough to expel any remaining fluid from the vagina. The douche pan is removed, the vulva and groins thoroughly dried with wool swabs, and if necessary a sterile pad applied. The mackintosh and towel are removed and the bed remade.

Soluble pessaries, containing penicillin or a sulphonamide, or stilbœstrol to increase the protective acid reaction of the vagina may be ordered, and should be inserted when the patient is in bed at the end of the day. A tray is taken to the bedside with a right-hand or disposable glove, or a finger stall with a cape, a pad and the pessary which has been checked with the prescription. The patient is asked to lie on her left side with buttocks at the edge of the bed, and the pessary introduced with the gloved hand along the posterior vaginal wall into the top of the vagina. Its position is important; it is useless simply to put it inside the vaginal orifice.

Painting the vagina with an antiseptic like Bonney's blue may be required, and the following articles will be needed:—

    Receiver with sponge-holding forceps and gauze-covered swabs
    Sims' speculum and lubricant
    Gallipot of required antiseptic
    Pad
    Mackintosh and towel
    Gloves
    Light

The bed is screened, the clothes adjusted and the patient lies on the left lateral or Sims' position with the mackintosh or towel beneath the buttocks, and her shoulders covered. The light is adjusted so that the nurse is afforded a clear view of the vulva, and the speculum lubricated and inserted. The speculum selected must be one that gives a good view of the vault of the vagina, and Sims' is excellent The cervix and anterior fornix are easily accessible, and the posterior vaginal wall must be gently retracted until the posterior fornix can be adequately treated. A swab held in the forceps is dipped in the antiseptic, and the top of the vagina thoroughly painted. The lower part is painted as the speculum is withdrawn, and the pad is supplied to prevent soiling of the clothes.

All these vaginal treatments call for neatness, gentleness, a knowledge of local anatomy, and a sympathetic insight into the patient's reactions to them. Descriptions in a text-book can give the technique involved, but cannot match the value of assisting an experienced nurse at the patient's bedside.

CATHETERIZATION

Catheterization of the urinary bladder is much less commonly performed than it used to be, because the dangers attached to its performance are better known. Even with the most careful technique, there is a high risk of introducing organisms into the bladder, and from here infection may ascend the ureter to the kidneys, causing pyelitis. Complete eradication of such an infection may be very difficult, and there may be recurrences which over the years may lead to destruction of kidney tissue and even eventually uræmia. Even if infection is confined to the bladder, cystitis can cause much misery to the patient.

The nurse knows that when she is performing a surgical dressing she must only allow sterilized equipment and lotions to come in contact with the wound, because her hands cannot be rendered sterile. The swabs and the catheter must be handled with forceps.

Catheterization may be performed in the gynæcological ward for the following reasons.

(1) To empty the bladder before operation. The bladder is closely related to the upper part of the anterior vaginal wall, and can easily be injured during pelvic operations. Catheters for this purpose are often inserted in the theatre rather than in the ward.

(2) To empty the bladder after operations on the anterior vaginal wall, or extensive pelvic operations. Micturition is often inhibited after such operations, and if the bladder becomes distended the stitch line may be disrupted. An indwelling catheter such as a Foley is used, and since it may have to remain in place for a week, the risk of bladder infection is high.

(3) To relieve retention of urine. Measurement of the amount of urine obtained is obviously important. If the retention is chronic, the nurse may be required to withdraw 200 ml. or so of urine, and to leave the catheter in place, closed with a spigot that can be released at intervals.

(4) To ascertain the residual urine, which means the amount of urine remaining in the bladder after the patient

thinks she has emptied it. Catheterization for this reason is used as rarely as possible.

(5) To obtain a specimen for identification of organisms, and their sensitivity to antibiotics. This is not now a common reason for catheterization; the bacteriologist will usually accept a *clean specimen*. The meatus and the inner surfaces of the labia are thoroughly cleaned and dried, and the labia held apart while urine is passed into a sterile container.

Procedure. If the patient is seen in a clinic, the vulva and inner surface of the thighs is well washed with soap and water. This may also be needed in the ward, but can be omitted if local toilet has been performed recently.

These articles are needed:—

> 2 pre-packed sterile catheters, size 7 or 8
> 2 drapes
> 3 gallipots
> 1 kidney dish
> Wool and gauze swabs
> 2 handling forceps (French, or similar)

} sterile

Clinical sheet
Cetrimide or Savlon
Sterile KY jelly
Measuring jug, or sterile specimen jar according to need
Bag for used swabs, drapes and disposables
Bag for used instruments

The sterile articles may be autoclaved together as a catheter pack, and if so they are wrapped in a paper towel which can be used to cover the trolley top and provide a sterile working surface.

Screens are drawn round the bed, and the patient told about the treatment to be performed. If she has not experienced it before, she is assured that it is painless. She lies on her back, with not more than two pillows under her head, and the assistant turns the bedclothes down to knee level. A clinical sheet is slipped beneath the buttocks. If an assistant is available, she prepares the patient while the operator arranges her trolley. The upper parts are covered with a blanket or bedjacket, the patient is asked to flex her knees and abduct her thighs and a lamp is adjusted to illumine the vulva.

PRE-OPERATIVE TREATMENT 37

She washes and dries her hands, and then opens her packs and arranges her equipment. Cetrimide or savlon is poured into a gallipot, catheter jelly is put into the other gallipot. Five wool swabs are wrung out of the cleaning lotion with forceps, and laid in a gallipot ready for use. A catheter is removed from its sterile pack with forceps, the eye end is dipped in lubricant, and the catheter put in the kidney dish. Again using forceps, the two sterile towels are arranged, one over the pubis, and one over the right thigh. The kidney dish is lifted with handling forceps, transferred to the palm of the free hand and placed on the bed between the patient's thighs. Care must be taken not to contaminate the interior of the dish.

The labia majora are cleaned with a downward stroke with moist swabs held in forceps. Two gauze swabs are used to separate the labia minora so as to expose the meatus

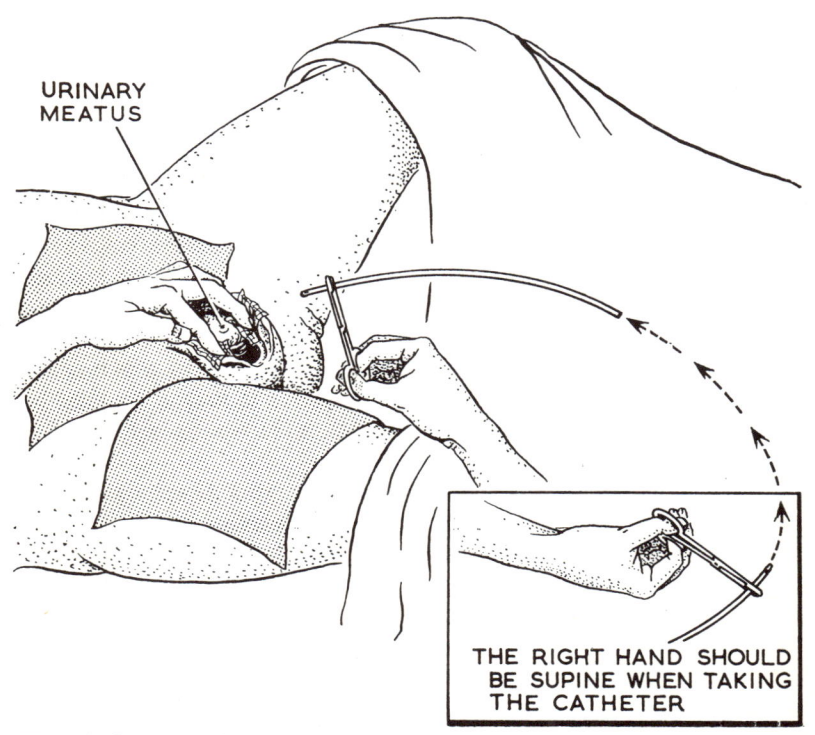

FIG. 16. Correct position of the right hand allows unimpeded view of the vulva

fully. The gauze swabs are held under the first and second fingers of the left hand to keep the labia apart. The meatus is now cleaned with the remaining swab, used with a downward motion once only. The meatus must be seen and identified confidently before attempting to pass the catheter, and there is no doubt that for a student nurse this is the most difficult part of the procedure. The clitoris and vagina are easily found, and in most cases the urethral orifice can readily be seen between them, but difficulty may arise if the anterior vaginal wall has descended, or if an operation has been performed on the vagina. Assisting an experienced operator is of the greatest value in learning how to identify the meatus in such cases, and the gynæcological ward sister should give her juniors every opportunity of seeing her methods.

Once the meatus is seen, the catheter is taken with forceps 4 cm. (1½ in.) from the eye end. The other end is left in the kidney dish, or dropped into a sterile jar if a specimen is required. The eye end of the catheter is lubricated, passed into the meatus, and advanced gently until urine begins to flow, which is when about 5 cm. (2 in.) of catheter has been passed. In some cases the urethra is elongated, and further passage is needed. This is often noted if catheterization is needed during labour.

When the flow stops, the patient is asked to cough to ensure that the bladder is empty, and the catheter is removed. The vulva is dried with the sterile drapes. The patient is thanked for her cooperation and the bed remade If a specimen has been taken the jar is labelled and sent to the laboratory. If not, the amount withdrawn is measured and recorded.

Self retaining catheters. These are used if they are to remain in the bladder. The most common type is a Foley, which has a balloon just behind the perforated tip. It is passed with the balloon collapsed and this is then inflated via the side tube. Water is used, to give more stability to the catheter, and this must be sterile in case the balloon ruptures inside the bladder. This is especially liable to happen if liquid paraffin is used instead of jelly as a catheter lubricant. The most commonly used type is that holding 5 ml.

If a Foley catheter is being passed, the additional articles required are a sterile 5 ml. syringe, and (for some types) a

PRE-OPERATIVE TREATMENT

no. 12 needle and sterile water. When the catheter is in position, the syringe is charged with water, the needle-mount pushed into the end of the side tube, and the balloon filled. There is a self-sealing device that prevents the water running out.

Bladder infection is common if an indwelling catheter is in use. Nitrofurantoin 100 mg. three times a day is often ordered to prevent this. The nurse should ensure that the vulva is kept quite clean, and the catheter, which will readily become encrusted by dried urethral secretion. This must be removed daily with swabs soaked in cetrimide. A good fluid intake is desirable to keep up an adequate urinary flow.

The bacteriologist is usually willing to accept a clean specimen of urine for culture. The meatus and the inner surfaces of the labia are thoroughly cleaned, the labia held apart while urine is passed into a sterile container. If a mid stream specimen is required, the first few millilitres are passed into a separate container, and discarded.

CHAPTER 4
POST-OPERATIVE CARE

WHEN the nurse receives her patient after operation, she is told the nature and extent of the operation performed and any other relevant information. This would include such points as the presence of abdominal drainage tubes; if there is a pack in the vagina; whether a catheter has been left in the bladder, and how it is to be managed; if any special difficulty was experienced at operation, and if any particular complication is to be feared. If intravenous fluids are being given she should know their nature, and the rate of administration. She accompanies the patient back to the ward, walking at the head of the trolley where she can see that the airway is satisfactory, and can support the jaw if necessary.

In the ward the patient's bed has been prepared with clean linen, and well warmed. The pillows are beside the bed ready for insertion when consciousness is regained, and on the locker are a vomit bowl and towel, and a tray with mouth gag, spatula, sponge-holding forceps and gauze-covered swabs. These may have been sent to the theatre with the patient, and will be put on the locker after her safe return on the trolley. A thermometer is at hand, and any special equipment that may be needed. For instance, it may be that an indwelling catheter will be in the bladder, and that it is the surgeon's practice to allow this to drain continually at first. A sterile Winchester or presterilized plastic bag (e.g. Uribag) will be needed, a sterile glass connection and an adequate length of rubber tubing in a sterile dish. If an antiseptic lotion is used, it must be measured, and it will not be possible to see the character of the urine that is draining.

If an electric blanket has been used to warm the bed, this is switched off and removed. Hot water bottles must be taken out of the bed of an unconscious patient, if these have been used. The patient is laid in the bed, on her side, and a warm blanket drawn over her. Before covering her with the rest of the clothes, dressings are briefly inspected, the nurse assures herself that there is no vaginal loss, and if necessary removes the spigot from the catheter and connects it to the tubing and jar, securing the tubing against displacement by a restless patient. The operation socks and outer theatre gown can be taken off if the condition is satisfactory, and the bed made up.

The temperature, pulse and respiration rate are now taken, and while doing this the nurse notices her patient's colour and whether the skin is dry or moist. Sweating is not an indication of overheating unless the temperature is normal and the colour rosy. If sweating occurs in a patient with a subnormal temperature and poor colour, it is because the skin is too cold to evaporate the normal insensible perspiration from it. The nurse dries the face with a towel, keeps her warmly covered, may raise the foot of the bed on blocks, and prepares to keep close observation on her patient, who is suffering from surgical shock, and will need the treatment given in the section on shock below.

The nurse remains with her patient until consciousness is restored and danger of respiratory embarrassment is past. If an artificial airway is in position it is not removed until movements of the mouth indicate that the swallowing reflex has returned. There are three main causes of difficulty in respiration:—

A. The tongue is relaxed and is obstructing the glottis. It occurs in a patient deeply unconscious, lying on her back, or in one who has had the artificial airway removed too early. The head should be turned to one side and the jaw supported forward. If necessary the gag is inserted in the corner of the mouth and the tongue depressed with the spatula. A nurse should never attempt to insert a spatula between the front teeth if they are clenched or they may be damaged.

B. Mucus is obstructing the airway. The mouth is opened in the way described, and a sponge-holder and swab is gently used to clear the back of the throat. Often breath-holding and congestion of the face indicate that vomiting is imminent, and every care must be taken that the head is kept to one side, lest vomitus be inhaled. This danger is not a theoretical one, and it is most likely after an emergency operation, if an anæsthetic has been administered to a patient with a full stomach.

C. Spasm of the glottis is a much less common but more serious condition. It is most often met after a short anæsthetic with pentothal. It is most likely to occur just as the patient is moved into bed, and the respiration ceases, because the vocal cords are in apposition. The head and neck should be extended, and the foot of the bed raised. If breathing is not at once resumed a message should be sent to the anæsthetist, and oxygen supplied with a suitable mask. A sterile 5 ml. syringe, No. 14 hypodermic needle and three 1 ml. ampoules of nikethamide are prepared, and it may be necessary to begin artificial respiration. When the anæsthetist arrives the nurse fills the syringe if he decides to give nikethamide by intravenous injection. Spasm of the glottis is only dangerous if it is not immediately recognized and promptly treated.

When the swallowing and cough reflexes have returned, a pillow is put under the head and the period of danger to the airway is over. There are many post-operative discomforts and complications that may happen, and which can be prevented or require treatment. Some of them are common to all surgical patients and some are especially associated with gynæcological work.

(1) Post-operative Vomiting

Severe post-operative vomiting should not be a common feature after modern anæsthesia, being unusual if it continues for more than an hour or two. A mouth wash and a clean bowl should be provided each time it is necessary, and if the vomited material is mucoid, a glass of warm sodium bicarbonate solution, a drachm to a pint, may hasten its removal. In a proportion of patients, vomiting is caused by morphine given pre-operatively, and if vomiting is troublesome, it is best not to give this drug after operation as it may only contribute to the difficulty.

A plain biscuit along with some fluid that the patient fancies, such as tea, is often effective, or a salty drink like Bovril meat extract may be tried. In severe vomiting drugs such as avomine, fentazin or phenergan may be used.

There is a certain functional element about post-operative vomiting in some patients, who associate the unpleasant complication mentally with all operations.

POST-OPERATIVE CARE

Sympathetic but firm reassurance is important in the early control of what may become occasionally a serious event, leading to dehydration and loss of chloride.

Severe or prolonged vomiting will require intravenous replacement of the fluid and chloride lost together with aspiration of the stomach through an indwelling Ryle's tube. Continued vomiting may be an indication of a more serious condition, like paralytic ileus (p. 50) or intestinal obstruction.

(2) Shock

Shock is nearly always the result of excessive blood loss and is not a marked feature except in a few operations such as Wertheim's hysterectomy, and other severe procedures for malignant growth. It is usually seen immediately on return from the theatre, but may be delayed for some hours, and is marked by these signs.

The temperature is subnormal and the skin feels cold and moist to the touch. The pulse volume is reduced and feels thready, and this is a much more important observation than the rate, which may be fast or slow, while irregularities of rhythm may be noticed. The respiratory movement is less than normal and the rate reduced. Estimation of the blood pressure shows a fall from the normal region of 120/80 mm. of mercury, and it may be difficult to record a diastolic pressure at all. The colour is poor, a hint of cyanosis in the pallor producing an appearance usually referred to as "livid." Restlessness may be shown if she is not deeply unconscious.

The surgeon may be aware of his patient's condition and have ordered the appropriate treatment, but if it develops after return to the ward he should be informed immediately. The foot of the bed should be raised and the patient kept warmly covered but not actively heated. There is a natural desire by the nursing staff to warm a patient who looks and feels so cold, but overheating may cause more fluid loss from the skin, and bring the blood to the surface where it will not only deprive the vital organs of the blood they need, but allow further heat loss and delay recovery. Hot water bottles are especially dangerous; pressure from even a warm bottle may cause a burn to devitalized tissues. If the patient is restless, morphine 10 mgm. is usually ordered.

If shock is severe, intravenous infusion will be needed, and if hæmorrhage in the theatre has contributed to the shock, blood is the obvious choice. It is cross-matched with the patient's blood, and it will be an important duty of the nurse to see that it continues running into the vein. Plasma or a plasma substitute may also be used, and has the advantage that grouping is not needed, while the protein in these solutions maintains the osmotic pressure of the blood.

Rest is most important to the patient with surgical shock. Constant observation is needed, but it should be remembered that taking the blood pressure too frequently is disturbing, and little information can be gained from it that cannot be seen from a ten-minute pulse chart, which involves no disturbance at all.

Oxygen with a mask at a rate of 6 litres per minute may be necessary if the pulse and colour indicate the need for it, and is beneficial to any patient suffering from shock.

With treatment on the lines indicated the shock should begin to abate, as will be seen by the improving colour and pulse volume and the rising blood pressure. **Failure to do so should give rise to the suspicion that some other** complication is involved, and the most common one is bleeding. If it is taking place from the vagina it will soon be noticed, but if it is taking place into the peritoneal cavity it can be diagnosed by clinical observation only.

(3) Hæmorrhage

This is a fairly common occurrence in gynæcology, being one of the most serious major complications. It is important that the nurse be able to recognize promptly its signs and symptoms and know what has to be done.

The first reaction of the body to an acute blood loss is to maintain the blood pressure and the pulse volume by a constriction of the arterioles. If bleeding continues this mechanism suddenly alters, the blood pressure drops rapidly, and the patient passes quickly into a profound and serious state of shock.

A patient who is losing blood rapidly is white, without at first the cyanotic tinge that is present in shock. The temperature is low and the pulse volume reduced while the rate slowly increases. Respiration is punctuated by sighs and yawns as oxygen lack begins to take effect, progressing to a gasping rhythm styled " air hunger." She feels faint and thirsty, complains that she feels as though she is sinking through the bed, and watches her attendants with an anxiety that is characteristic. If the pulse is taken at five-minute intervals a steady rise in rate will be shown. It is important, however, not to think that because the pulse has taken an hour to rise from 80 to 90 that it will take another hour to rise to 100. A change may come very suddenly, so that in the course of a few minutes she may become cold and pulseless, with a diastolic blood pressure too low to record. It must be obvious that in the post-operative period this picture will be obscured by the effects of the anæsthetic, and will not be seen in its typical form. If a patient is apparently suffering from shock, the surgeon must be informed at once; if she does not improve with rest, fluids and a suitable posture, he will suspect that concealed bleeding is taking place.

Gynæcological hæmorrhage can occur at any time. PRIMARY bleeding happens at the time of injury or operation. The nurse may see it in the theatre, or in such cases as incomplete abortion. The control of bleeding at the time of operation is the responsibility of the surgeon. REACTIONARY hæmorrhage occurs within a few hours after operation, when the patient's condition is improving and the blood pressure rising. A severed vessel, not noticed at the time, begins to bleed, or a ligature slips from a vessel that has been tied. If the bleeding is into the peritoneal cavity, it is the observations of the intelligent nurse and her alertness in interpreting them that will reveal the condition. A change for the worse in the temperature, pulse and blood pressure, or a deterioration in the condition of a patient for whom no anxiety was felt on her return from the theatre, will mean that the surgeon must be informed. If abdominal examination confirms that bleeding is taking place into the abdominal cavity, she will go to the theatre to have the bleeding point secured, and will probably need transfusion.

The bladder is catheterized, clots removed from the vagina, and the bleeding point, which is usually visible, is secured. If the origin of the blood loss cannot be seen, the vagina is tightly packed with sterile gauze soaked in hibitane or another suitable antiseptic cream.

If the hæmorrhage is from the vagina, there is no difficulty in deciding what has happened. If the bleeding point cannot be seen (and usually it cannot), the bladder is catheterized, clots are irrigated away from the vagina, and it is tightly packed with dry sterile gauze. It would be exceptional for this to be performed in the ward when theatre facilities were available. To be really effective it needs an anæsthetic, the lithotomy position, and the rigid asepsis that only the theatre can provide.

SECONDARY hæmorrhage is an infrequent but still alarming complication of vaginal operations, and is always due to sepsis. The facilities for controlling sepsis should make this kind of bleeding progressively rarer. The vagina is not sterile and is very vascular so that the conditions for secondary bleeding are present. It occurs typically between the eighth and fourteenth days, and is seldom quite unheralded. A little irregularity in the temperature and some rather offensive vaginal discharge are danger signs, and steps should be taken to cure the infection that may cause the bleeding.

At first a small or warning hæmorrhage may be noted, and must be reported to the doctor. One or two days later, sudden and severe secondary bleeding may occur, and medical help must be called at once. If the patient is not in bed she must be put there, with one pillow under her head and the foot of the bed raised. If the nurse feels agitated, she must on no account let her patient sense it, but remain with her, encouraging her by her calm competence, and indicating that all will be well. If she receives instructions to give morphine she will administer it at once, which will do much to quieten the patient's fears. A mackintosh and large pad are placed beneath the buttocks, and if frequent inspection is necessary the bedclothes may be divided for convenient access. Any soaked dressings are saved for inspection, and the pulse taken at short intervals and unobtrusively. The patient should not be left alone.

The treatment depends on the severity of the bleeding. A hot vaginal douche may occasionally be ordered, and if so the trolley previously described should be prepared, with six pints of normal saline at 118° F. (3 litres at 48° C.). A layer of Vaseline petroleum jelly should be applied to the perineum and adjacent areas over which the solution will flow, lest burning should occur, and a rubber catheter size 14 is better than a rigid douche nozzle. Douching, however, is disliked by most surgeons, and should never be used unless it is specifically ordered, and a vaginal pack will have to be used in a serious case.

This is, of course, best performed in the theatre under an anæsthetic, since it is not easy in a frightened restless patient to do it effectively in the ward. Isolated instances will occur, however, in which there is unavoidable delay in obtaining medical assistance, and in which the bleeding is alarming and progressive, and in such a case it is clearly the duty of the nurse to apply the appropriate treatment in the ward. The bladder should be catheterized, and a vaginal pack inserted which will render micturition impossible. Sterile gauze rolls, sponge-holding forceps, Sims' speculum and a good light are necessary. If the nurse has to insert the pack herself, she should place her patient in Sims' position, insert the speculum, and fill the vagina as closely as possible, pressing the gauze firmly into the vault of the vagina with the forceps.

(4) Pain

Pain at the operation site will need treatment by drugs. Soon after recovery from the anæsthetic a suitable injection will be given, and it must not be withheld until pain is severe and the patient anxious and alarmed, since timely administration may mean that less sedative is needed later. Morphine 10 mgm. will allay fear as well as relieving pain, while pethidine is very effective for gynæcological patients, and 50 or 100 mgm. may be given by intramuscular injection. In most instances it will be necessary to repeat the injection, in order to secure a comfortable first night, and after that injections may be no longer needed. Codeine or aspirin mixtures are useful and effective, and can be given in quantity sufficient to keep the patient free from pain, e.g. tabs. Codeine Co. B.P.C. 2 p.r.n.

Those who have wounds in the vagina and perineum often suffer discomfort from swelling and tension of the sensitive surrounding areas, and everything possible should be done to relieve it, including careful toilet, and if necessary the removal of any sutures that are cutting into the tissues.

Pain is also associated with bladder complications and abdominal distension, the treatment of which is described under the appropriate headings.

(5) Chest Complications

Post-operative pulmonary infections are not unduly frequent in gynæcological wards. Comparatively few women are heavy smokers, while midline incisions in the lower abdomen do not inhibit the breathing movements to any great extent. Morphine, which is an important respiratory depressant, is used less post-operatively than in some surgical specialities.

Pre-operative breathing exercises are a great help in preventing post-operative chest complications. Those which may occur are as follows:—

(1) **Broncho-Pneumonia.** The patient may be a middle-aged woman who had some chronic bronchitis associated with a cold or cough before operation. On the second day she complains of phlegm on the chest which the pain in her wound prevents her from coughing up. The temperature rises to 37°–37·8° C. (99°–100° F.), and the respiration rate increases to 22 or 24 a minute. There is flushing of the face, mild sweating, and, often a tight feeling in the chest. These early signs are not dramatic, but treatment must be begun at once, or by the next day the nurse may see a flushed ill woman whose temperature is 38·3°–38·9° C. (101°–102° F.), and whose breathing gives audible signs of mucopurulent secretions in the lungs. If she has an abdominal wound, it should be supported firmly on each side while she coughs up any secretion, and the physiotherapist can clap the back of the chest. Steam inhalations four-hourly will help to loosen secretions. The doctor may order an expectorant, such as sodium chloride mixture, and treatment by an antibiotic such as penicillin or tetracycline is usually started immediately. A specimen of sputum should be sent to the laboratory to ascertain the sensitivity of the organisms to antibiotics so that the administered drug is shown to be correct, or may be altered if required. The fluid intake should be kept high, and an improvement can usually be expected in twenty-four hours.

(2) **Massive or Lobar Collapse.** If respiratory movements are inadequate, or the secretion is tenacious,

mucus may fail to be expelled from a bronchus and may block its lumen, preventing the passage of air to and from the lung. The air present in the lobe of lung supplied by this bronchus is soon absorbed, so that the lobe becomes collapsed and airless. This is marked by a sudden rise in temperature, pulse and respiration rates on the first or second day after operation, and the patient has a characteristic feeling of unease and distress. No other complication produces this sudden upward swing of all three rates so soon after operation, and without any abdominal signs. The houseman on examining the chest confirms that an entire lobe of lung is collapsed and dull.

The patient must be at once encouraged to cough up the mucus that is obstructing the bronchus. She may be laid on the unaffected side with the head lowered, and percussion over the airless lobe is vigorously undertaken. As a last resort suction through a bronchoscope is used, but the nurse will rarely see a patient in whom it is needed. She will be struck by the rapid fall in temperature, pulse and respiration rates that follows re-expansion of the lobe, and should thereafter see that her patient practises deep breathing frequently and takes fluids freely.

(3) **Pulmonary Infarct.** This will be discussed below in connection with pulmonary embolism.

(6) Abdominal Distension

This used to be a very common accompaniment of gynæcological operations, and the fact that it is still frequently seen should not lead the nurse to regard it as inevitable or unworthy of attention, since to some patients it may be the most miserable feature of the post-operative period, or may in some cases be the prelude to a more serious condition.

A completely fluid diet should not be given without special reason, for the introduction of simple solid foods will help to prevent flatulence. Neither, on the other hand, should bulky carbohydrate meals be given. Unless the operation is one for repair of the vagina, a mild aperient can usually be given on the third evening after operation, and a suppository on the fourth morning, when distension is usually at its worst. A suppository is not likely to be effective if given earlier; unless some peristalsis is established, it will afford no relief. The passage of a rectal tube, to get rid of flatus, sipping hot peppermint water, or the administration of codeine or aspirin mixture are all of help in tiding the patient over a rather unhappy time, which tends naturally to cure itself about the third or fourth day when normal bowel movements are restored.

After a vaginal operation, special management of the bowel is necessary, and will be described under the detailed account of the management of these patients (p. 128).

Exceptionally, distension may become severe, with a rising pulse rate and vomiting, and the serious condition of PARALYTIC ILEUS is diagnosed. Peristalsis ceases, and from a functional point of view there is intestinal obstruction. Some cases are due to peritonitis, and a full course of antibiotics will be begun if there is any suspicion of infection, but in some cases there is no apparent cause. These patients require the utmost medical and nursing care.

The stomach must be kept empty, both to allow it to regain its tone and to prevent the distressing vomiting, so a Ryle's tube is passed transnasally to remain in the stomach, or a Miller-Abbot or Cantor tube which should pass onwards into the small intestine may be preferred. Continuous suction may be applied, or in the case of a Ryle's tube aspiration with a 50-ml. syringe is done often enough to prevent vomiting. This fluid must be accurately measured, since the loss of fluid and electrolytes must be replaced by intravenous infusion. Morphine 10 mgm. may be ordered six hourly, and estimation of the serum chloride and potassium will decide what electrolytes should be given.

Some of the nursing points that are important are to keep the patient comfortably supported, to treat the dry mouth at frequent intervals, to keep the fluid balance chart accurately, and to maintain the intravenous infusion at the rate ordered. The pressure points should be regularly treated with as little disturbance as possible, and the patient's morale and courage maintained. A decrease in the distension, a falling pulse rate and the passage of flatus indicate that this grave condition is responding to treatment.

Intestinal obstruction of a mechanical kind may also occur after any operation on the abdomen. If there has been extensive removal of pelvic organs, a loop of small intestine may become adherent to a raw area and produce obstruction. Severe colicky pain occurs, followed by vomiting, the amount of which is in excess of the fluid intake. The vomit is at first stomach contents, then becomes bilestained, and later opaque and brownish, with a characteristic intestinal smell. The temperature is low, the pulse rate shows a progressive rise, the tongue is dry, and the expression drawn and anxious. If the vomiting is promptly reported to the surgeon, the patient will not reach the serious condition described, but will undergo laparotomy for the relief of the obstruction as soon as gastric suction and intravenous infusion have been begun. Her treatment afterwards is along the lines indicated above for paralytic ileus.

(7) Urinary Complications

Many gynæcological patients on admission have urinary symptoms such as frequency, dysuria and stress incontinence, whilst patients with prolapse are especially prone to have a urinary infection. It is, therefore, not surprising that many patients suffer post-operatively from some trouble connected with micturition, since about 15% of all admissions suffer from a urinary tract infection.

URINARY TRACT INFECTION

Infection in the urinary tract may affect the kidney (pyelonephritis); the ureter (pyelitis); the bladder (cystitis); or the urethra (urethritis). Cystitis is the commonest urinary tract infection, and may be present prior to admission. If so, it must be treated and eliminated prior to operation.

Infection may have been present in the bladder on admission, and if so it should be cleared by antibiotics before operation. Stagnation of urine within the bladder leads to infection, while catheterization, however scrupulous the technique, carries the same risk. It is, therefore, obvious that if normal micturition is not established after operation, retention of urine must not be left untreated, but neither must catheterization be too hastily undertaken, since both may cause infection. A high fluid intake together with a prophylactic course of sulphacetamide g.1, q.1.d. for two days then g.1, b.d. for two days are useful measures, as is nitrofurantoin, 100 mgm. q.i.d. for four days.

RETENTION OF URINE

This is one of the commonest complications, especially after vaginal operations, when the close proximity of the operation site may lead to œdema of the bladder wall. It is particularly common following operations for the cure of stress incontinence of urine. Most surgeons keep a self-retaining catheter in the bladder following vaginal repair operations for at least forty-eight hours, because normal micturition is unlikely to be established immediately after operation. If a patient does not pass urine after operation, the resultant retention is painful and demoralizing. The passing of a catheter will be uncomfortable for the patient and the recent operation may make the urethral meatus difficult to find. It is, therefore, incumbent on the nurse to ensure that the bladder does not become distended, and if an indwelling catheter is used to see that it is draining freely.

Adequate relief of pain is a big step towards establishing normal bladder function, because a woman who is tense and miserable is unlikely to succeed in emptying her bladder. Within twelve hours of operation she is given a warm bedpan, comfortably supported and no suggestion is made that there may be any difficulty. Failure should not be commented on, but a bedpan should be offered an hour or two later, and if the bladder is not then emptied, simple methods of suggestion may be tried to evoke the reflex. Running nearby taps, and pouring a pint of warm water over the vulva into the bedpan are well known. After many operations, most surgeons would allow the patient to sit on a commode beside the bed twenty-four hours after operation, and this is usually successful. If the patient is still unable to pass urine, a catheter must be passed, and in this case a prophylactic course of nitrofurantoin should be started immediately or a course of sulphacetamide together with potassium citrate and hyoscyamus mixture.

It cannot be stressed too strongly that a post-operative

record of the frequency of micturition and of the amount passed must be kept accurately, and the fluid intake measured. Such a chart may indicate quite clearly how the urinary system is functioning. For instance, in a woman who has been suffering from retention of urine, the passage of small amounts of urine at frequent intervals may mean that she is suffering from RETENTION with OVERFLOW. This dangerous condition must be relieved by catheterization as soon as it is diagnosed. The catheter should be left in situ on continuous drainage for at least forty-eight hours. Some surgeons may prefer catheterization to be repeated three or four times in twenty-four hours until the amount of residual urine left in the bladder after micturition is no more than an ounce or two.

By far the commonest cause of failure to pass urine is retention, due to œdema, reaction, or mechanical causes but occasionally it may be due to SUPPRESSION—that is, no urine may be reaching the bladder from the kidneys.

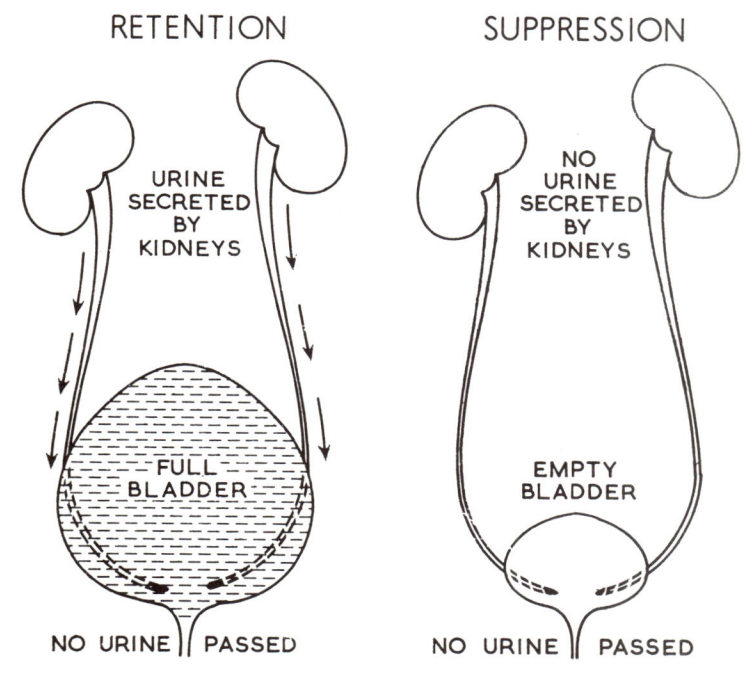

FIG. 17. Failure to pass urine may be due to suppression or retention and these must be distinguished.

The patient feels no desire to urinate, and no discomfort in the bladder, and the passage of a catheter confirms that it is empty. This very serious condition can be caused by bilateral ligature or section of the ureters, a catastrophy which is not impossible in operations for malignant disease. It demands urgent urological investigation and relief of the obstruction by appropriate surgical measures, e.g. the removal of a ligature, implantation of the proximal end of the cut ureter into bladder or sigmoid colon, or bringing it out on to the skin of the abdominal wall, or even nephrostomy, i.e. draining the kidney temporarily through the loin.

INCONTINENCE OF URINE may occasionally be seen after operation. The patient might be one who had undergone a Wertheim's hysterectomy, which involves stripping the ureters of their surrounding tissue in the pelvis. This sometimes leads to sloughing of a part of the ureter, so that on the tenth day a watery discharge appears from the vagina, which on investigation proves to be urine. Such a uretero-vaginal fistula will have to be dealt with surgically, and in the meantime the nurse must prevent the skin becoming sore by the use of a barrier cream, and by frequent changing of the vulval pad. The patient's morale must be sustained by assurance that the setback is a temporary one.

A fistula resulting in incontinence of urine may also occur between the bladder and vagina following total abdominal hysterectomy or any vaginal operation. The causes and treatment of vaginal fistulæ in general are discussed on p. 153.

To sum up, urinary troubles are by far the commonest post-operative complication. The surgeon endeavours to prevent them by gentle handling of structures at operation, the nurse by strict asepsis during catheterization, and by intelligent and accurate observations and records. The antibiotics are powerful weapons in preventing and treating infection.

(8) Thrombosis and Embolism

Clotting within a vein, or phlebothrombosis, is one of the commoner of the major post-operative complications in gynæcology. It is of two types. One of these can be seen not infrequently in veins that have been the site of intravenous infusions, especially if these have been long continued, and dextrose saline alone has been used. The vein wall becomes irritated by the solution, and an aseptic inflammation results which produces clotting within the vessel. The patient complains of pain, a little fever occurs, and the vein can be seen and felt as a tender red swelling in the rather œdematous limb. This condition is troublesome, but not serious, and heat in the form of kaolin poultices will usually relieve the symptoms. The clot is firmly adherent to the vein, and as the inflammatory reaction subsides the lumen becomes recanalized.

Thrombosis of a different and much more serious nature may, however, occur in the legs, especially the calves, in a normal vein with no inflamed wall to anchor the clot in position. Such thrombosis is due to stagnation in the blood flow, and the following factors may contribute to it:—

(1) Prolonged recumbency.
(2) Pressure on the calves, either on the operating table or in bed.
(3) Low blood pressure, as in shock.
(4) Anæmia.
(5) Pelvic operations. These appear to carry a special risk, as a similar tendency is noted after prostatectomy in men.
(6) Inadequate respiratory movement. The action of the diaphragm on the inferior vena cava is of importance in helping the return of blood to the heart from the legs.
(7) Fear is believed to increase the clotting power of the blood.

Any of these factors may operate in gynæcological surgery unless the medical and nursing staff are vigilant.

Signs and Symptoms. Three or four days after operation slight evening pyrexia may, but does not always, occur. Some tenderness may appear in one or both calves, of which the patient may complain spontaneously, or which may be elicited by pressure on the calves. There may be some swelling, which becomes more obvious if the clot extends into the thigh. Should it spread into the common femoral vein, gross œdema occurs, and the condition is known as "white leg." Once a fairly common complication in both gynæcology and obstetrics, it is now very rarely seen.

The danger of this kind of thrombosis is that such a clot may detach, pass upward in the blood current through the inferior vena cava, and through the right ventricle to the pulmonary artery. This is PULMONARY EMBOLISM, and by cutting off the blood supply to one or both lungs it may cause sudden death in a most tragic way.

Prevention of Thrombosis. Remembering the factors that cause thrombosis, it is possible to prevent it occurring in many cases. Breathing exercises, correction of anæmia and a moderate amount of mobility are practised before operation. Careful arrangement of the patient on the theatre table can avoid pressure on the calves, and modern surgical technique can avert shock in many patients. Pillows beneath the knees after operation are not allowed, and movement of the legs should be encouraged. Getting the patient out of bed a day or two after operation is helpful when it is possible, and the nurse should see that the patient stands on her feet, as the movement of dorsiflexion is especially helpful to the circulation in the calves. When making the bed the nurse must feel the calves and ask if they are comfortable (not if they are painful) and any tenderness is at once reported to the medical officer.

Drugs are available which decrease the coagulability of the blood and so prevent the growth of the thrombus. The only drawback to their use in a surgical patient is their tendency to start bleeding at the operation site, and it has already been seen that hæmorrhage is a well recognized complication in gynæcological cases. Where no such risks exist, or where they are thought less important than the fear of pulmonary embolism, the following regime is a typical one.

Heparin 10,000 units is given by intravenous injection six-hourly on the first day, and a course of phenindione is also begun. 100 mgm. may be given twice on the first day, 50 mgm. twice on the second, and the subsequent dosage will be governed by the prothrombin time of the blood, which is maintained between 20% and 30% of the normal. Much variation in anticoagulant technique exists in

POST-OPERATIVE CARE

different hospitals, especially in the amount of mobility ordered for the patient.

Pulmonary Embolism. The signs and symptoms

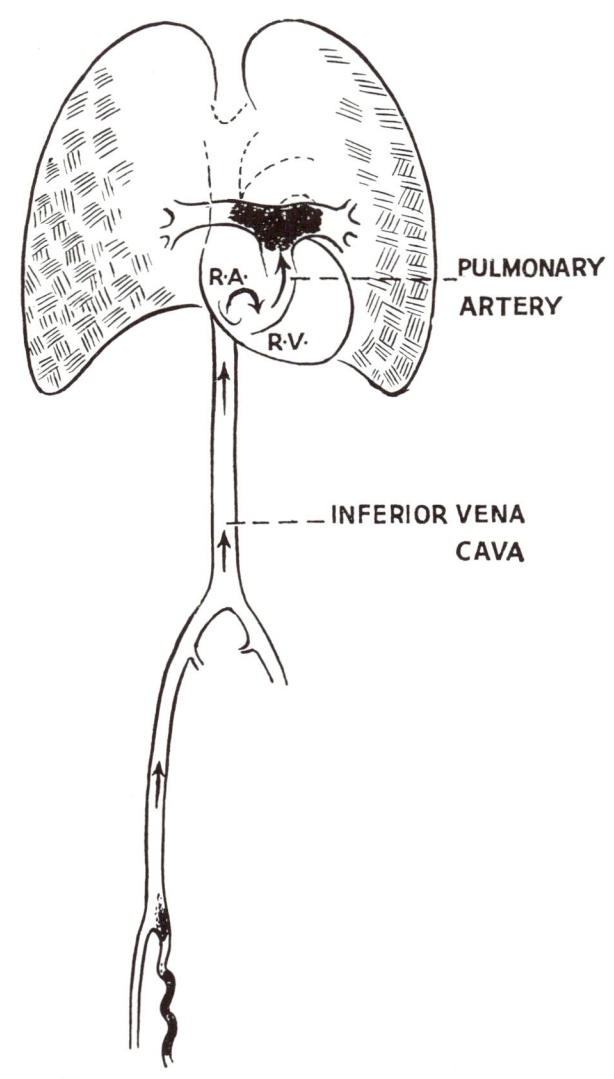

Fig. 18. Massive Pulmonary Embolism. A diagram showing the path of the embolus from the leg veins through the inferior vena cava to the right heart and to the pulmonary artery. The branches to both lungs have been blocked, and an embolus of this size would be rapidly fatal.

associated with this severe circulatory disaster depend on the size of the embolus. It may be that the clot which has broken loose is several inches long, and nearly as thick as the nurse's little finger. As it passes through the heart it causes strong reflex stimulation of the vagus nerve, and the resulting wave of peristalsis makes the patient ask urgently for a bedpan. Before the nurse can reach her, the embolus may have blocked the main pulmonary trunk, and the patient dies instantly. If it is not quite so large, she collapses into a state of extreme shock. The pulse is imperceptible, the skin livid and cold, and the temperature falls. Consciousness may not be lost, and in this serious emergency the nurse must not allow her alarm to be seen.

The house surgeon is summoned at once, and screens drawn round the bed. Absolute rest is essential, and no attempt should be made to lay the patient flat, but oxygen at 8 or 10 litres per minute should be given with a mask. When the doctor arrives he will probably order morphine 16 mgm., and may want to give 10,000 units of heparin intravenously, so the necessary sterile syringes and needles should be prepared.

The patient's condition may remain critical for some time, and such cases must always be considered as candidates for an operation to remove the clot after thoracotomy. This formidable operation is now used more frequently, and may be the only way of saving the patient's life. It entails moving a desperately ill woman to the anæsthetic room in her bed, which may prove too much for her. Absolute rest, morphine and oxygen are otherwise the best ways of dealing with it. Nikethamide by intravenous injection, or even adrenalin into the heart may be tried, as last resorts, but, in the absence of operation, those who need such remedies are unlikely to survive.

If the embolus is a small one, it blocks the blood supply to an area at the periphery of the lung, and the damaged area whose blood supply is thus interrupted is called an INFARCT. The patient experiences a sharp pain in the chest over the part, which continues and becomes sharper with each inspiration as a pleurisy develops over the infarct. The temperature rises after a few hours, and the breathing is rapid and shallow. Later some blood-stained sputum may be coughed up.

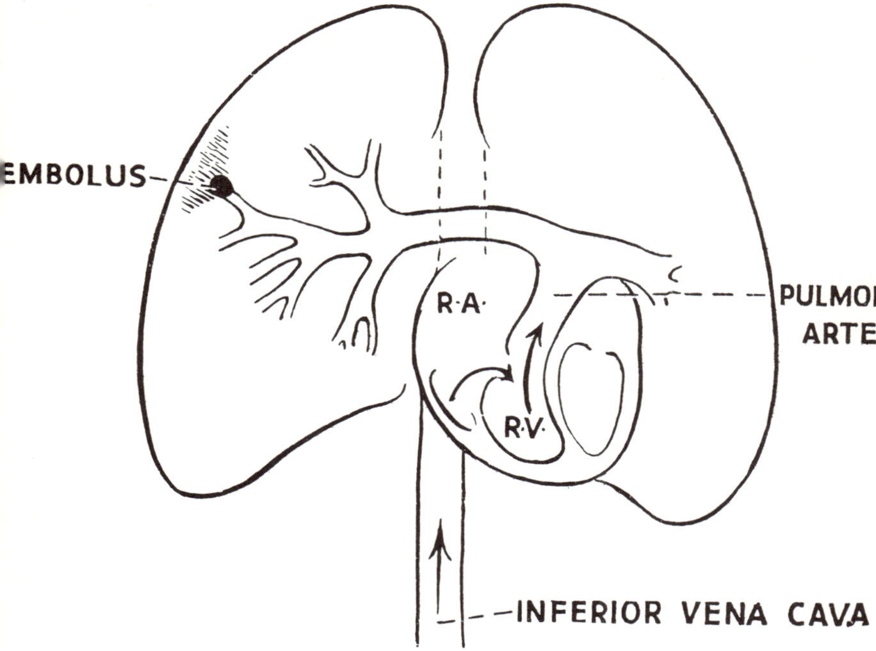

FIG. 19. Pulmonary Infarct. An embolus has entered the right pulmonary artery and blocked a small branch. The part deprived of its blood supply (infarct) is represented by the shaded area.

Anticoagulant therapy is usually begun, as a small embolus may be the herald of a much larger one. Kaolin poultices will help to relieve the pain in the chest. The surgeon has to decide how much mobility the patient is to be allowed, and the decision is not an easy one. Strict immobilization will allow extension of the clotting, while too much movement may encourage the breaking loose of more clots. The tendency to-day would be to give gentle leg exercises in bed at once, and to get the patient up when the temperature was normal and the prothrombin time satisfactory. The nurse must make sure that she understands the surgeon's wishes and follows them exactly.

Other measures have been used for patients with venous thrombosis in the legs in whom pulmonary embolism is feared. Tying the common femoral vein would seem a certain way of cutting the pathway from the clot to the heart, but in some cases further clotting may occur above the ligature and cause embolism. In such instances the inferior vena cava has been ligated as a life-saving measure, and it is surprising that this heroic operation leaves the patient with comparatively little or even no œdema of the legs. Fortunately, while venous thrombosis is common, few patients develop pulmonary embolism, but if a nurse encounters a fatal case, it is quite likely to be when she is working in the gynæcological wards.

(9) **Wound Sepsis.** Abdominal wounds ordinarily heal cleanly and without difficulty, but occasionally tension and redness in the incision indicate infection, and if this appears to be centred around a particular stitch, the stitch should be removed. Small collections of pus may become evident in the subcutaneous tissues, and the insertion of a pair of sinus forceps into the incision line is usually sufficient to drain these, and sodium sulphate dressings and kaolin poultices will hasten their dispersal.

A hæmatoma, or collection of blood within the tissues, may occur within the abdominal wall, and should be evacuated. It may become infected if allowed to remain, or will eventually discharge. A 5 or 10 ml. syringe and a No. 1 needle may be used to aspirate the fluid from the swelling.

Infection of vaginal and perineal incisions is much more common and in moist areas like these (exposed, in the case of the perineum, to gross contamination) it is impossible entirely to eradicate sepsis. Much can be done, however, to minimize it by careful vulval toilet, repeated each time a bedpan is used, until stitches are out and healing complete. The following are required:

1 litre jug of lotion at 40·5° C. (2 pints at 105° F.)
(normal saline or hibitane.)
Plenty of sterile swabs, and a pair of sterile forceps.
Sterile pad.
Receiver.
Clean bedpan.

The patient is settled in a recumbent position on a bedpan with the thighs flexed. The jug is taken in the right hand and lotion poured first over the vulva then particularly over the introitus and perineum, holding the labia minora apart with the first and second fingers of the left hand. Without moving the left hand, the jug is set down and a swab taken with the forceps. The area is now thoroughly and meticulously cleaned, each swab being discarded as it is drawn over the perineum. Every scrap of mucus and secretion is swabbed away, and if the stitches are of catgut any that are sloughing may be removed. The area is left perfectly clean and dry. This procedure should be continued until all stitches are out and the perineal stitch line is well healed and dry. If stitches other than catgut are used, they can usually be removed about the eighth day.

(10) Burst Abdomen. Formerly bursting of the abdominal wound after the stitches had been removed was not uncommon, and it was for instance often expected after operation for cancer of the stomach. These patients were in fact those whose diet had been severely restricted by their disease, and who were suffering from vitamin C deficiency. It is not now often seen. If there is any cause to suspect such a deficiency, 500 mgm. of ascorbic acid can be given by intravenous injection before operation, and the routine use of 25 mgm. twice a day by mouth before

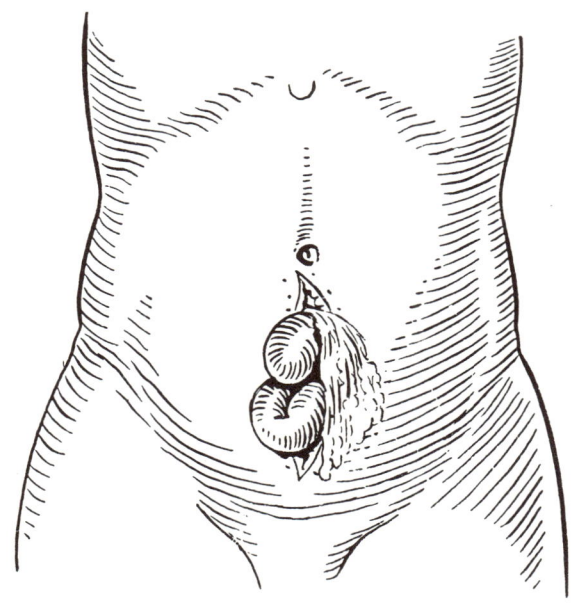

FIG. 20. Burst Abdomen. Small intestine and omentum are seen escaping from the wound.

and after operation for all patients undergoing major surgery is advisable.

Bursting of the abdominal wound usually occurs soon after the stitches have been removed, and it is usually associated with infection in the wound. Chronic cough and abdominal distension may contribute to it. The patient feels a sharp pain and inspection of the wound reveals that part, or rarely all of it, has opened. Coils of intestine may be seen beginning to protrude, or may not be visible. A message is sent to the surgeon, and a sterile towel wrung out of hot saline is laid over the area, and wool and a binder applied over it. Secondary suture will be undertaken in the theatre and the prognosis is good, alarming though this complication appears when first seen.

All the post-operative complications described above can be to some extent prevented, though no amount of vigilance will abolish them altogether. These complications mean not only distress and pain to the patient, but cause a longer stay in hospital which is expensive, and prevents another woman in need of treatment from occupying the bed. If the nurse's part in such prevention is examined, it will be seen that her biggest contribution can be made by acquiring a scrupulous aseptic technique and being alert to observe and report the earliest signs that trouble is impending.

CHAPTER 5

DISEASES OF THE OVARY

Anatomy. The ovaries are oval in shape, 4 cm. long, 2 cm. wide, and 1·5 cm. thick. They are described as lying on the side wall of the pelvis, but they enjoy a greater freedom of position than this, and may be found anywhere in the true pelvis. The Fallopian tubes encircle them above, and the open ends of the tubes overhang them. Each ovary is attached to the uterus near the origin of the tube by the ovarian ligament, and to the pelvic wall by the infundibulopelvic ligament, which carries the ovarian blood vessels, and the lymphatics which drain to glands on

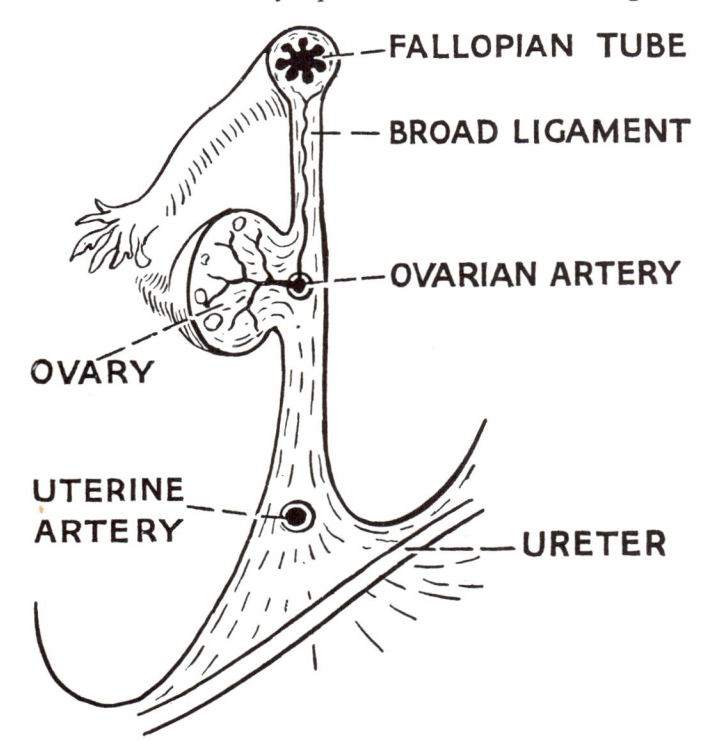

Fig. 21. Diagrammatic section through the ovary and neighbouring structures.

the posterior abdominal wall in the region of the renal arteries. Before puberty the ovaries are small and inactive, but throughout the reproductive period they undergo the regular activity described on p. 6. Their removal means not only that ovulation and menstruation ceases, but that the patient is deprived of endocrine glands of great physiological importance.

Ovarian Tumours

In gynæcological practice ovarian tumours of many varieties are encountered. In fact the ovary provides the richest source of pathological material of any organ in the body. The majority of these tumours are cystic; that is, swellings filled with fluid, and most are innocent, but some are highly malignant.

In view of the fact that the ovary contains thousands of immature ova capable in favourable circumstances of producing all the complex elements of the human body, it does not seem surprising that a range of tumours can be formed in connection with them.

Besides cysts arising from the egg apparatus, there is a further number derived from the connective tissue of the ovary, and another important group arising from epithelial elements.

Another interesting class of ovarian tumours is that in which the cells of the growth produce an active endocrine secretion, sometimes feminizing, and more rarely masculinizing. The feminizing tumours can cause bleeding from the uterus before puberty and after the menopause. The masculinizing variety stop menstruation, and in time they produce a striking change in the patient's appearance, causing hirsuties, masculine body conformity and deepening of the voice. Their timely removal may restore menstruation and procure a reversion to the original sexual type. Both of these tumours are potentially malignant. Finally, the ovary is all too frequently the site of primary and secondary cancer.

The pathology of the ovarian cysts is not of great importance to the nurse, who wants to know the symptoms that bring her patient to hospital, the treatment she is likely to be offered, and her prognosis. Those described here are the common varieties.

Cysts of the Egg Apparatus, or Follicular System

If a Graafian follicle fails to rupture, its fluid contents are retained, and a small cyst develops in the ovary. Such swellings are not new growths in the real sense, but retention cysts, and they are spoken of as FOLLICULAR CYSTS. CORPUS LUTEUM cysts are cysts which form in the corpus luteum (i.e. after ovulation has occurred). They do not usually cause symptoms, and regress spontaneously, but occasionally they may secrete enough progesterone to suppress menstruation for several weeks, thus giving a false impression of pregnancy. Rupture of the cyst may result in hæmorrhage into the peritoneal cavity, which may be sufficiently severe to require laparotomy and ligation of the vessel in the ovary. They are usually small, and may give rise to no complaints. A follicular cyst may, however produce œstrogen, and give rise to heavy and prolonged uterine bleeding. (See Metropathia Hæmorrhagica, p. 99.) These swellings, unlike all other ovarian cysts, do not as a rule need operative removal, and many indeed are discovered by chance during laparotomy for some other condition.

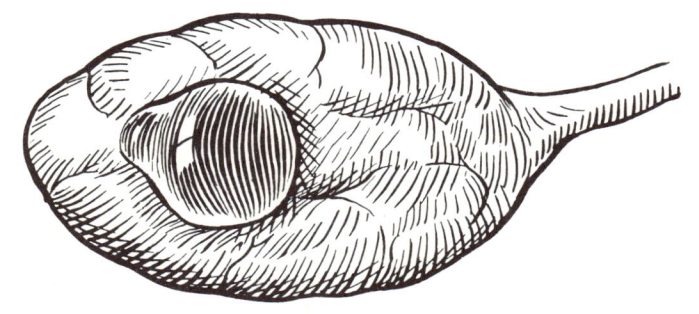

FIG. 22. Follicular cyst of ovary.

Endometriomata, or Chocolate Cysts

Both these names are descriptive, one of the apparent origin, and the other of the contents of these common cysts. The cyst wall resembles the lining membrane of the uterus, and they contain dark altered blood. The lining of the cysts obeys the endocrine stimulus of the ovary just as the lining of the uterus does, and at each menstrual period some bleeding takes place into the cavity of the cyst. This blood becomes thicker and darker as time goes on, and the cyst slowly enlarges, but rarely exceeds 15 cm. in diameter, and is usually less than 5 cm. in diameter. Their origin was in doubt; the old theory depended on the observed fact that during menstruation blood may regurgitate along the Fallopian tube into the peritoneal cavity. It was suggested that living endometrial cells present in this blood might in some circumstances settle on the ovary and grow into chocolate cysts. Endometriosis (i.e. the presence of chocolate cysts) may occur also in the uterine walls, pouch of Douglas, the uterine ligaments, and more rarely in the bladder, bowel, or even more distant situations.

The clinical picture is of a woman in her mid-thirties, often childless, who suffers from increasing pain, and (in half the cases) excessive loss during menstruation. The pain is due to the distension of the cyst with blood, or to adhesions caused by scarring adjacent to the cyst.

Simple Serous Cyst

This is a single thin-walled cyst full of watery fluid. It is not usually more than 10 cm. in diameter, can arise at any age, may cause pressure symptoms, and should be removed when diagnosed.

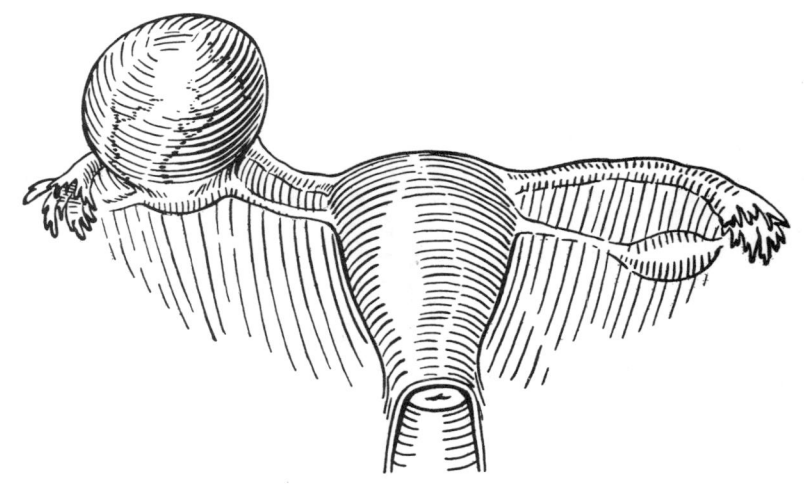

FIG. 23. Simple Serous Ovarian Cyst.

Papilliferous (Papillomatous) Cyst

The wall of a papilliferous cyst is studded with warty excrescences projecting into the cavity. If these papillæ

DISEASES OF THE OVARY 67

grow, as they sometimes do, through the cyst wall, they may spread into the peritoneal cavity, causing ascites. Yet in

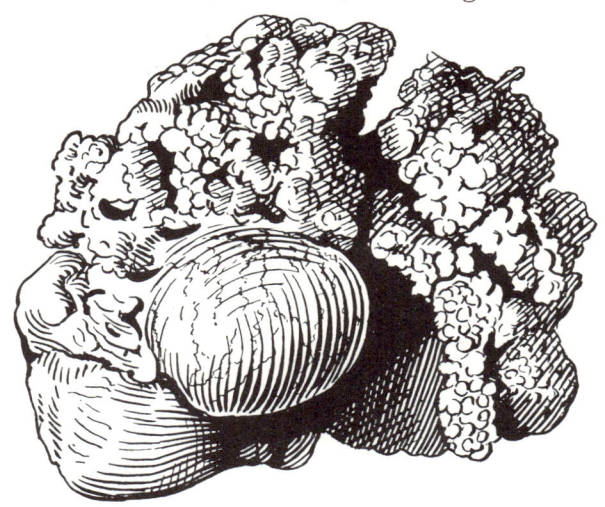

FIG. 24. Papilliferous Cyst. The papillæ have penetrated the cyst wall and are growing into the peritoneal cavity.

spite of this surface activity, many are innocent, though all are potentially malignant. If the parent cyst is removed, the outlying papillæ may disappear, provided the parent tumour is benign.

Pseudomucinous Multilocular Cyst

This, the commonest ovarian new growth, is remarkable for its ability to grow to great dimensions. Cysts as big as a full-term uterus are common, and growths have been recorded of 100 kg. and over. Their name describes them adequately; that

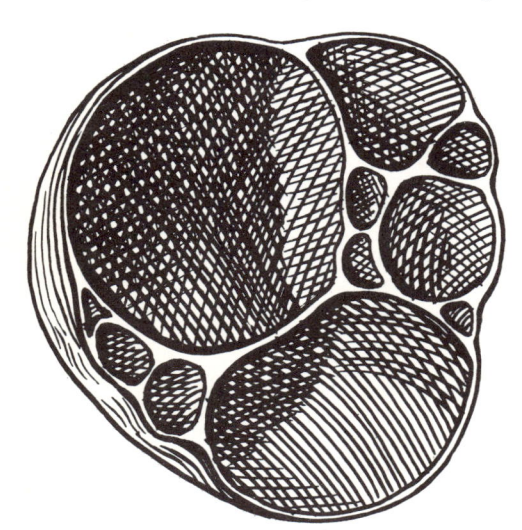

FIG. 25. Section through a Multilocular Ovarian Cyst.

68 MODERN GYNÆCOLOGY FOR NURSES

is, they are of many compartments, filled with thick glairy material. Fifty per cent. of them contain a node of malignancy; hence the importance of surgical advice on all ovarian swellings, and the removal of all those greater than 5 cm. in diameter.

Dermoid Cyst

Dermoid cysts capture the imagination because of their bizarre contents. They seldom grow larger than a cricket ball, and contain sebum, and such structures as hair, teeth, cartilage, brain, bowel and even thyroid tissue, which may

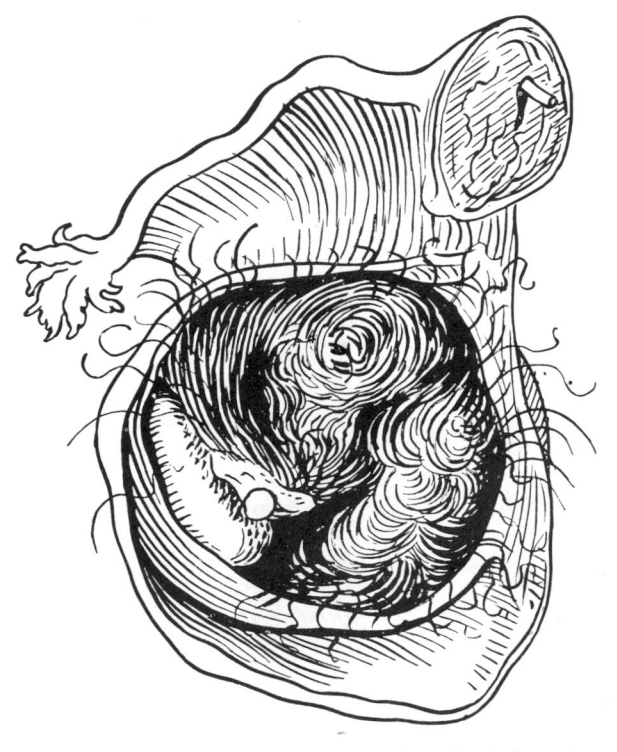

FIG. 26. Dermoid Cyst. The cyst contains hair and a tooth, and the cavity would be filled with sebaceous material.

become active and cause thyrotoxicosis. They occur most frequently in young women between 20 and 30, and are sometimes diagnosed at an antenatal examination without having previously produced any signs of their presence.

DISEASES OF THE OVARY

They are sometimes detected by an X-ray disclosing teeth in the pelvis. Most are innocent, but occasionally they become malignant.

Fibroma of Ovary

This is an innocent, solid, fibrous tissue growth. Its peculiarity is that sometimes ascites and pleural effusion arise in connection with it (Meigs' syndrome), and may lead to a diagnosis of malignant disease being made by a surgeon who feels the hard growth in the distended abdomen. The peritoneal and pleural fluid will disappear once the fibroma has been removed.

A number of other kinds of tumours occur more rarely, and a nurse who encounters a patient with one of these and wants to know more about it should refer to an advanced text-book.

Carcinoma of Ovary

Carcinoma is, unfortunately, a common ovarian tumour. Primary cancer of the ovary accounts for 25% of ovarian neoplasms. If a cancer appears near the surface, as in the breast, where it is easily palpable, or if it interferes with some vital function, the surgeon has some chance of seeing it early when a cure may be effected. A carcinoma of

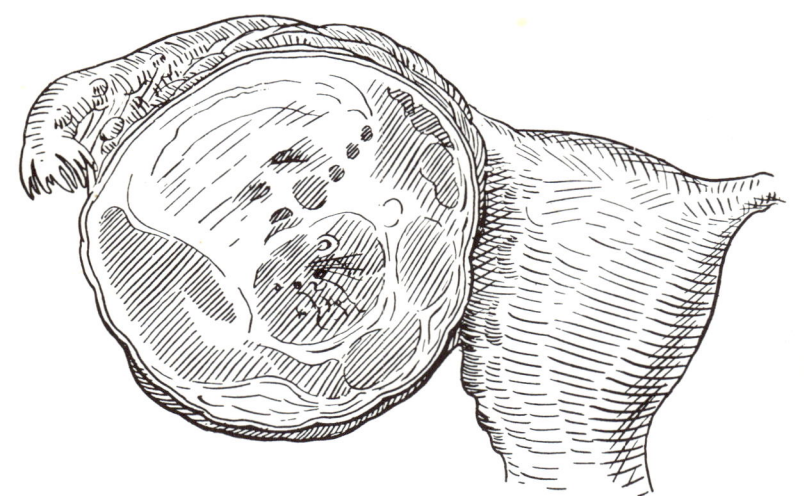

FIG. 27. Carcinoma of Ovary. The right ovary has been completely replaced by a solid malignant growth.

ovary falls into neither of these categories, and rarely gives rise to trouble until it has spread into the general peritoneal cavity, caused ascites, and therefore become incurable by surgery.

Secondary deposits in the ovary may result from a primary growth in the uterus, breast, stomach or bowel. Such secondaries grow very rapidly and usually outstrip the primary in size. They have a marked tendency to be bilateral. The surgeon who finds a hard fixed lump in an ovary makes a careful search for a primary growth elsewhere, since it would obviously be an error to submit a patient to an extensive pelvic operation for a growth which was only an incident in the spread of a completely different malignant disease.

Signs and Symptoms of Ovarian Tumours

Innocent ovarian tumours often cause very few symptoms. These can be considered as follows:—

(1) **Increasing Girth.** If the growth is large enough to rise out of the pelvis, the patient may notice abdominal swelling. If the tumour is a big pseudomucinous cyst this swelling may be considerable.

(2) **Changes in Menstruation.** Cysts of the follicular system are the only ones likely to cause such changes. Amenorrhœa is uncommon. Even patients with big bilateral cysts will menstruate normally as long as some ovarian tissue remains. Granulosa-cell tumours, the feminizing tumours mentioned above, cause post-menopausal bleeding.

(3) **Pressure Symptoms.** These occur very frequently. Pressure of the swelling on the bladder prevents it filling to the normal extent, so that frequency of micturition results. Indigestion is quite a common complaint, and occasionally constipation occurs, though most ovarian cysts are too soft to obstruct the bowel. Large tumours may cause shortness of breath, and palpitation may be experienced.

(4) **Pain.** Pain often amounts to no more than pelvic discomfort, and is only severe if some complication has occurred. Chocolate cysts may cause severe pain, especially before and during menstruation.

(5) **Cachexia.** If the tumour is large, even though it be innocent, much weight may be lost.

Symptoms of Ovarian Cancer

Carcinoma of the ovary rarely causes complaint until pain declares its spread into the peritoneal cavity. Ascites then soon follows, and œdema of the legs; the complexion becomes pale and emaciation is marked. A hard swelling can be felt on one or both sides. The most distressing feature of the later stages is the grossly distended abdomen produced by the ascites.

Complications

The presence of an ovarian cyst renders the owner liable to certain complications:—

(1) **Torsion.** If the cyst grows from a pedicle, twisting of the stalk may take place, which first compresses the veins in the pedicle, causing engorgement of the cyst and

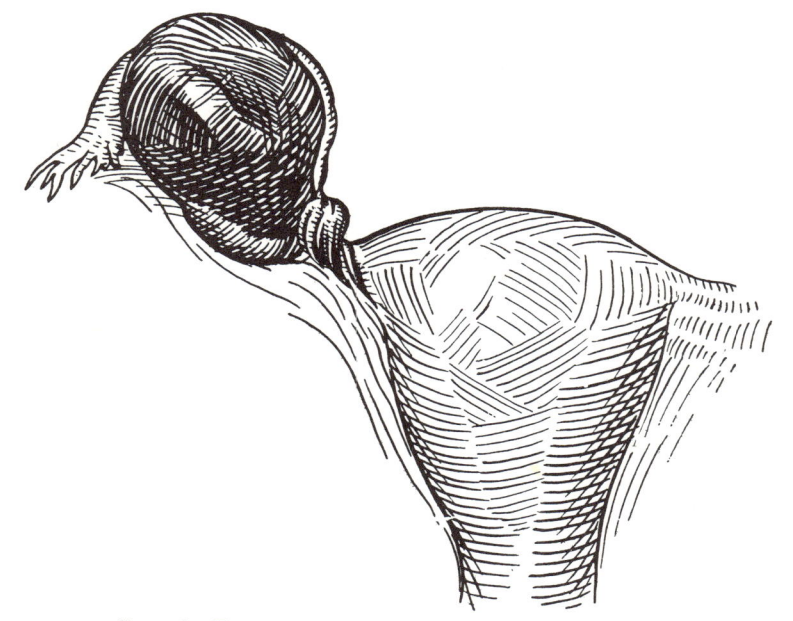

Fig. 28. Torsion of the pedicle of an ovarian cyst.

intense abdominal pain. Torsion is often accompanied by shock, shown by a subnormal temperature and weak pulse, and vomiting is usual. Dermoid cysts are particularly liable to this accident.

(2) **Rupture.** A cyst may rupture either spontaneously

or as a result of trauma such as a pelvic examination. A sharp pain is felt at the time of rupture, and is replaced after a short time by the severe pain of pelvic peritonitis as the contents of the cyst cause peritoneal inflammation.

(3) **Infection.** Infection of a cyst occasionally occurs, especially if it is adherent to the intestine.

(4) **Malignancy.** Follicular, simple serous and chocolate cysts do not undergo malignant change. About 25% of papilliferous and pseudomucinous cysts become malignant. However, as one in every four ovarian growths is said to be a cancer, this possibility must influence treatment.

(5) **Obstructed Labour.** The presence of an ovarian cyst in a pregnant patient is dangerous, since the cyst may become impacted in the pelvis below the head of the baby and may prevent delivery.

Treatment of Ovarian Cysts

With the exception of the cysts of the follicular system all growths of the ovary should be removed. The cyst itself is completely excised (OVARIAN CYSTECTOMY or OVARIOTOMY). If possible any normal ovarian tissue is kept, since there is a tendency for these cysts to affect both sides and if one ovary is removed, the patient may present later with a cyst in the only remaining ovary. Sometimes, however, there is no possibility of conservation, and removal of the ovary (OÖPHORECTOMY) has to be performed. The opposite ovary and uterus should always be inspected while the abdomen is opened.

When chocolate cysts are present on both sides it is often difficult to decide the extent of removal necessary. If small cysts are left the patient may be no better, while the removal of all would entail the loss of both ovaries. The surgeon remembers that castration entails severe physical effects in a woman below the age of the menopause, and avoids it whenever he can.

Treatment of Carcinoma of Ovary

If a carcinoma of ovary is seen early enough to make operation feasible, the uterus and both ovaries should be removed, and a course of deep X-ray therapy to the pelvis considered. The unaffected ovary is removed because of

DISEASES OF THE OVARY

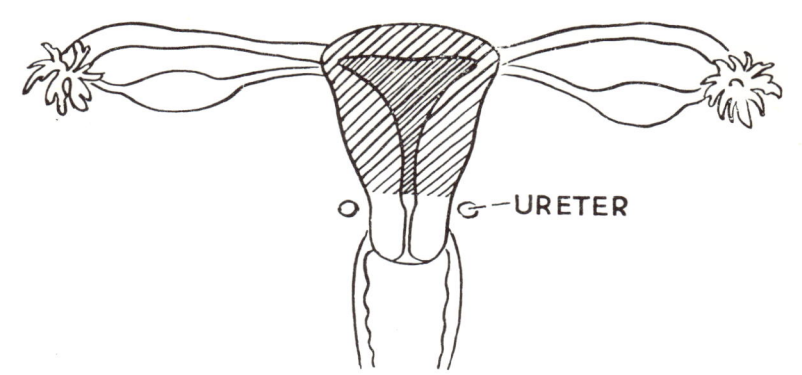

Fig. 29. Diagram to show the amount removed by subtotal hysterectomy.

the tendency of malignant ovarian growths to affect both ovaries, and the uterus is also removed because it may become involved in an extension of the growth.

This is a convenient place to explain the terms applied to removal of the uterus and its appendages. SUBTOTAL HYSTERECTOMY means the removal of the body of the uterus, leaving the cervix behind. This operation is used for some innocent growths of the uterus, and although safe

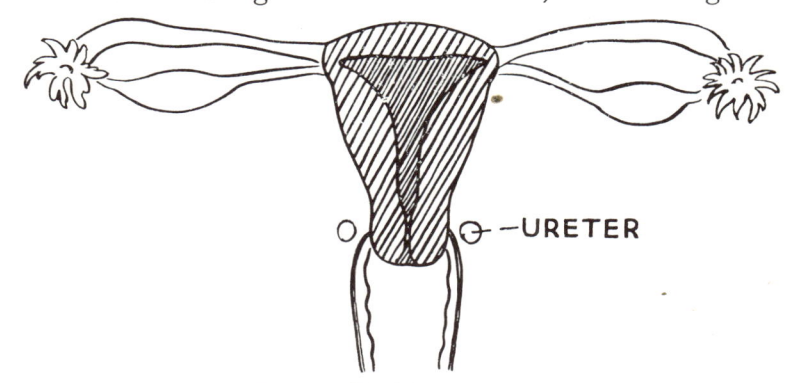

Fig. 30. Total hysterectomy.

and easy it is disliked by many surgeons because of the risk of cancer developing subsequently in the cervix. They consider TOTAL HYSTERECTOMY, or excision of the whole uterus, as a better operation. In malignant disease, the appendages must be excised as well—TOTAL HYSTERECTOMY with BILATERAL SALPINGO-OÖPHORECTOMY.

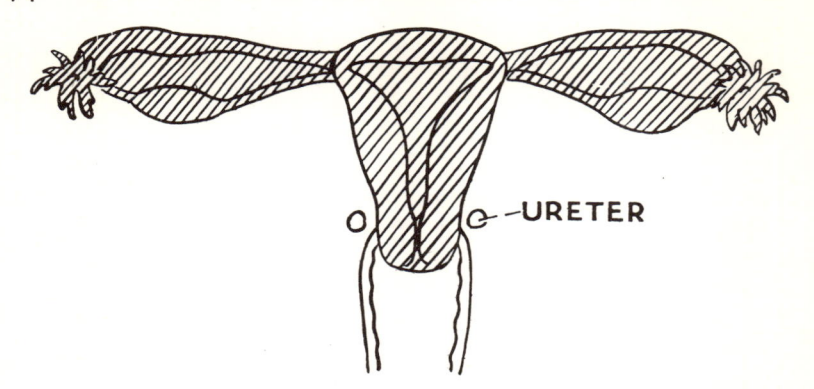

FIG. 31. Total hysterectomy with bilateral salpingo-oöphorectomy.

A still more extensive operation, WERTHEIM'S HYSTERECTOMY, is practised, especially for carcinoma of the cervix. Not only are the uterus and appendages removed, but the connective tissue around the uterus, the pelvic glands and the upper half of the vagina. Such a severe operation may cause surgical shock and a certain post-operative mortality.

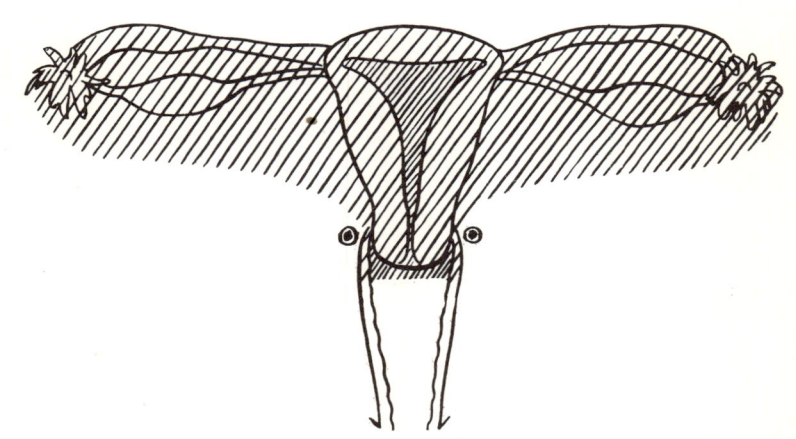

FIG. 32. Wertheim's hysterectomy.

If it is not possible to remove a malignant ovarian growth, X-ray therapy alone may be tried, but is not very successful. Severe ascites is the dominating feature clinically, and it is treated by paracentesis abdominis at the necessary intervals.

DISEASES OF THE OVARY

Paracentesis Abdominis

It is wisest to empty the bladder by catheter beforehand in order to avoid accidental puncture. A trocar and cannula is usually employed, or Southey's tubes are effective. A suitable sized tube is selected, prepared as in the diagram and sterilized in an autoclave. The cuff of rubber tubing is to slip over the cannula hole after the trocar has been withdrawn.

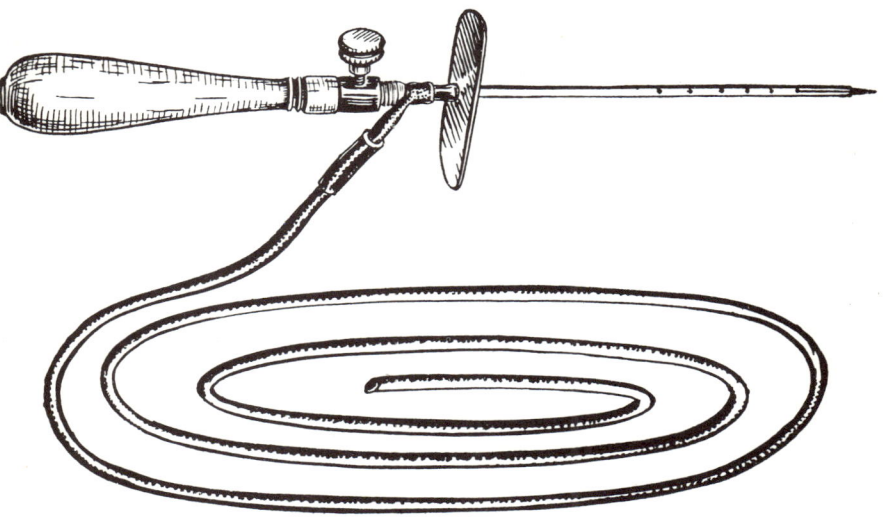

FIG. 33   Trocar and cannula.

Trolley

Sterile instrument tray with:—

    Trocar and cannula or Southey's tube prepared for insertion.
    Scalpel.
    Hypodermic syringe 2 ml. capacity and needles size 19 and 14.
    3 gallipots.

Sterile towels and swabs.
Pathological jar if a specimen is required.
Æther. Cetavlon. Spirit.
Procaine 2%.
Many-tailed bandage.
Tray with strapping, scissors, pins, clip.
Shawl or blanket.

Mackintosh and towel.
Winchester or drainage jar in a resection tray.
Receiver.

Procedure. When the bladder is empty, the patient is sat up against pillows, and told of the increased comfort that tapping will give. The nightdress is rolled up to the waist, the chest covered, the bedclothes folded down to the thighs and the mackintosh and towel put over them. The many-tailed bandage is placed behind the patient. The jar in its tray is put on the floor and the selected cleaning lotions poured out. The site chosen is to one side of the midline, half-way between the symphysis pubis and the umbilicus, and the skin is cleaned and the local anæsthetic injected. A small nick in the skin with a sharp scalpel facilitates the introduction of the trocar and cannula. The free end of the tubing is put in the jar, the instrument introduced and the trocar withdrawn, when fluid will commence to flow. Nurses often think that there is danger of puncturing the intestine, but in practice this does not occur because the bowel is movable and evades the point. Strips of plaster over the shield hold the tube in position and the tubing is adjusted to avoid leakage.

The abdominal binder is now firmly applied, and it may hold more firmly if a layer of wool is put underneath it. The clip is, if necessary, applied to control the rate of flow. This may be fairly brisk if the patient is used to tapping, but one should be cautious if it is the first occasion. The nurse remakes the bed, loosely tethering the tubing with a pin to the drawsheet. She remains with the patient until she feels that no reaction will take place. Some women feel faint as the abdominal pressure falls, and the best treatment is to tighten the binder, slow the flow a little and reassure the patient. A simple restorative like sal volatile may be indicated, but a reaction severe enough to necessitate calling the doctor and preparing a hypodermic stimulant is rare.

After clearing her equipment the nurse at frequent intervals returns to see her patient and inspect the level in the jar. The fluid withdrawn is measured and may amount to many litres before the cannula is removed and a collodion dressing applied to the puncture wound.

Radiotherapy

Radioactive colloidal gold in saline may be injected into the peritoneal cavity in the hope of limiting the ascites. The patients most suitable are those with multiple peritoneal seedling growths, but no large malignant masses. The effusion is tapped before the gold is introduced, and on return to the ward the patient must be turned systematically from side to side, from the recumbent to the prone position, and finally should have first the foot and then the head of the bed elevated. This ensures the distribution of the gold throughout the peritoneal cavity.

If tapping has to be performed within two weeks of injection, the fluid withdrawn is still radioactive and the isotope department should be consulted about its disposal. Nurses in wards where patients have radioactive substances on or in them should wear film badges to ensure that they are not receiving more than the permitted maximum of radiation.

Cytotoxic Drugs

Search is always being made for drugs that will cure or at least check the course of malignant disease. While none of those known to us at present has more than a temporary effect, there are some that are a valuable palliative measure in controlling symptoms. Unfortunately, the bone marrow is almost as susceptible to these drugs as new growths are, and a falling white cell count eventually indicates that treatment must be suspended. Development in this section of pharmacy is rapid, and newer drugs that are more effective and less toxic will certainly be produced. Many of those now in use are given chiefly for leukæmia or lymphadenoma, and the two described below are those which have some hope of improvement for those with neoplasm of the ovary or uterus.

Triethyl thiophosphamide ("Thiotepa") is given in these doses; 0·45 mgm. per kilo bodyweight intravenously for 4 days, or 0·9 to 1·8 mgm. per kilo bodyweight for injection into serous cavities. The results are not usually apparent for two or three weeks, and maintenance courses can be given.

Cyclophosphamide ("Endoxan"). The daily dose is 100–200 mgm. orally, or 200–400 mgm. by intravenous injection. It can also be injected into the peritoneal cavity. Nausea and vomiting, and temporary loss of hair can occur as transient side-effects. Therapy must be maintained indefinitely by the oral administration of 50–100 mgm. of cyclophosphamide. The white cell count is repeated frequently to ensure that the bone marrow is not being depressed too far.

Cyclophosphamide and other new cytotoxic drugs are being used with increasing frequency.

Nursing the Inoperable Patient

A great deal may be done by careful and imaginative nursing to reduce the patient's discomfort. The pressure points need regular treatment in this emaciated patient. The appetite will be diminished by the ascites, and the meals should be small in bulk and residue, and high in caloric value. Constipation is common, and if even a mild aperient like milk of magnesia or liquid paraffin causes discomfort, glycerine suppositories may be better. If the legs are œdematous, a cradle in the bed may give comfort, and a small pillow should be put beneath the ankles to keep the heels off the bed, and a support provided for the feet. Analgesics should be simple at first—aspirin, phenacetin or codeine mixtures, but morphine should not be withheld when these fail to control pain. Every endeavour should be made to alleviate any symptoms of which she complains.

Ovarian Dysfunction

Functional disorders of the ovary are common, and are chiefly manifest in deviations from the normal menstrual pattern. The account of these irregularities beginning on p. 96 should be consulted.

Inflammation of the Ovary

Infection of the ovary (oöphoritis) is not common except as an extension of inflammation from the Fallopian tube, and such tubo-ovarian infection is described on p. 84.

Virus oöphoritis sometimes occurs in girls who contract mumps after puberty. It is less common than the analogous condition of orchitis in boys, or perhaps is less easy to diagnose.

DISEASES OF THE OVARY

OÖPHORECTOMY FOR MALIGNANT DISEASE

When œstrogen starts being produced in quantity at puberty, the breasts, under its influence, enlarge and mature. Since normal breast growth is controlled by this ovarian hormone, it is not surprising that abnormal or malignant growth in the breast should also be sensitive to the presence of this œstrogen, and a great deal of work has been done in this field of endocrine treatment of carcinoma of the breast.

If surgery and radiotherapy fail to control a carcinoma of breast, secondary deposits usually enter the blood stream and form metastases in the lungs and bones. These secondaries can be influenced, sometimes dramatically, by such measures as bilateral oöphorectomy, though the exact way in which this œstrogen withdrawal acts is not directly understood. Such an operation may be effective even after the menopause, showing that œstrogen production does not entirely cease then. In other cases, the diametrically opposed treatment of administering œstrogen may also secure a remission. Cure does not appear possible by either of these methods.

Still more extensive operations are used in attempt to influence malignant growth by withdrawing endocrine stimulus. Bilateral adrenalectomy and removal of the pituitary gland are practised and further work on these major procedures is still continuing.

CLINICAL USES OF OVARIAN HORMONES

Difficulties arise in connection with treatment by the ovarian hormones because the natural hormones are not single substances, but contain several active constituents and the clinician in an attempt to make use of their different effects prescribes a range of synthetic drugs which resemble them in action. Varying results are obtained from the use of these substances in practice, and the list of approved and proprietary names is formidable.

Œstrogen

Natural œstrogen, or follicular hormone, is not a single entity but several hormones, of which œstradiol seems to be the most important. Œstrone and œstriol also occur in the body, but œstradiol and its derivatives which are made in the laboratory are the most widely used synthetic œstrogens.

These are active when taken by mouth, just as effective as natural œstrogen, and far cheaper. Stilbœstrol and ethinyl œstradiol are the ones most commonly prescribed, and hexœstrol and dienœstrol are also used. All are liable to cause anorexia or nausea when given in large amounts, and an adjustment of the dose or a change to another variety may be indicated.

Œstrogen may be prescribed for menopausal symptoms (p. 16), for senile vaginitis (p. 142), or vulvo-vaginitis in children. It is helpful in certain cases of functional uterine bleeding (p. 99), and is sometimes prescribed for primary amenorrhœa (p. 96). It is most useful in suppressing lactation, for instance when a baby has been stillborn, or in the treatment of a breast abscess. For many years œstrogens have been used for suppression of ovulation to control spasmodic dysmenorrhœa, and this action has recently been utilized in the production of the sequential type of contraceptive pill which contains 15 days of œstrogen followed by 6 days of progesterone.

One of its more unusual and successful applications is in carcinoma of the prostate gland in men. Decrease in size of the primary growth and of its secondary deposits in bone is often achieved by stilbœstrol, and years may be added to the patient's life. Soreness of the nipples is sometimes noticed as a side effect in men.

Progesterone

The corpus luteum hormone cannot be isolated in large amounts from ovarian tissue; it can only be made by a lengthy expensive process, and has to be given by injection. There are many different types of manufactured synthetic progesterones, which are powerful in action.

These synthetic progesterones have two main actions. Firstly they will suppress ovulation, probably by their action on the pituitary gland, and secondly, they induce and maintain the secretory phase of the endometrium. This action in suppressing ovulation is utilized in the " contraceptive pill." Progesterones are used in the treatment of some types of menstrual irregularity; in endometriosis; in threatened or habitual abortion; and in carcinoma of the body of the uterus. They may also be combined with œstrogen to treat patients with primary amenorrhœa.

CHAPTER 6

DISORDERS OF THE FALLOPIAN TUBES

THE Fallopian tubes are the passages by which the ova reach the uterus, and are 18 to 22 cm. long. It is usual to speak of the tube as having four parts.

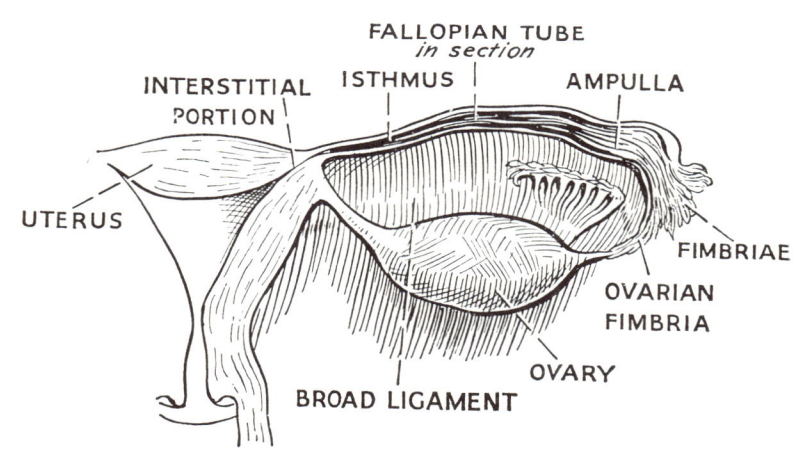

FIG. 34. Fallopian tube; its parts and relations.

(1) The medial end opens into the uterine cavity just below the fundus, so that the first part, or INTERSTITIAL portion, is that which lies in the uterine muscle, and is 1·5–2 cm. long.

(2) Next comes a narrowed portion, the ISTHMUS.

(3) The third part is the AMPULLA, and is the widest part of the tube.

(4) The abdominal opening of the tube is fringed with processes called FIMBRIÆ. One of these—the ovarian fimbria—is longer than the others, and is attached to the ovary.

Peritoneum is reflected from the bladder over the uterus and tubes, and down behind them to the pouch of Douglas in front of the rectum. The tube thus lies in the top of a double fold of peritoneum, the BROAD LIGAMENT.

This structure is of some importance in the pathology of the Fallopian tube, and contains many vestigial structures which may give rise to cysts. The abdominal ostium of the Fallopian tube opens near the side wall of the pelvis into the peritoneal cavity, so that infections of the uterus or tubes are able to cause peritonitis, which may remain localized in the pelvis, or become general.

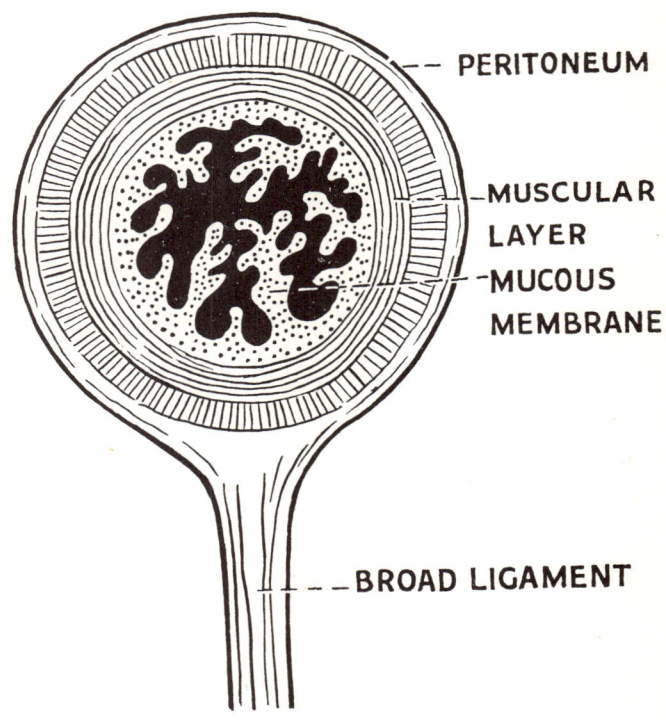

FIG. 35. Section through the Fallopian tube.

The wall of the tube is muscular, and its lining mucous membrane is ciliated, and thrown into ridges which in the ampulla are elaborate and complicated. The cilia maintain the flow of mucus from the ovarian to the uterine end, and the muscle wall is capable of peristalsis. Both these actions are increased by the influence of œstrogen, and so are most in evidence at the time of ovulation, when they facilitate the passage of the ovum to the uterus.

DISORDERS OF THE FALLOPIAN TUBES

The ovarian artery and the uterine artery both contribute blood to the tube, and this double blood supply is of the greatest importance in determining the reaction of the tube to infection. Gangrene of a tube is never caused by infection, whereas the appendix, with a single arterial source of blood, is prone to it.

INFECTIONS OF THE FALLOPIAN TUBE

Inflammation of the tube is SALPINGITIS, and such an infection may arise in one of three ways.

(1) The infection spreads upwards from the uterus, the lining of which is also infected (acute ENDOMETRITIS). Such a uterine infection is most likely when the mucosa is not intact—during menstruation, or following abortion or full-time delivery—and the organism is usually a streptococcus or staphylococcus.

Acute gonorrhœa (p. 159) may also spread from the cervix to the endometrium and thence to the Fallopian tubes.

Salpingitis is most commonly due to an ascending infection of this kind, and naturally tends to be bilateral.

(2) Infection may reach the tube from the peritoneal cavity. An inflamed appendix may give rise to salpingitis, in this way, and so may tuberculosis of the peritoneum.

(3) Blood-borne infections are rare but do occur. Tuberculosis may affect the tubes without any evidence of peritoneal infection, thus indicating that it has travelled by the blood stream from a primary focus elsewhere, usually in the lungs.

Pathology. Salpingitis may be acute, and if inadequately or unsuccessfully treated may become chronic. Tuberculous salpingitis is always insidious, and the infection is chronic when first seen.

Acute salpingitis may be a mild condition confined to the mucous membrane, with little constitutional upset. It may resolve completely or may result in adhesions between the delicate folds of the tubal mucosa, which may later have a serious effect on the patient's fertility.

In any case of salpingitis, the abdominal opening may become sealed by adhesions, and if the narrow interstitial part is also blocked, infected secretions accumulate within the tube which swells to some size. The ampulla is the

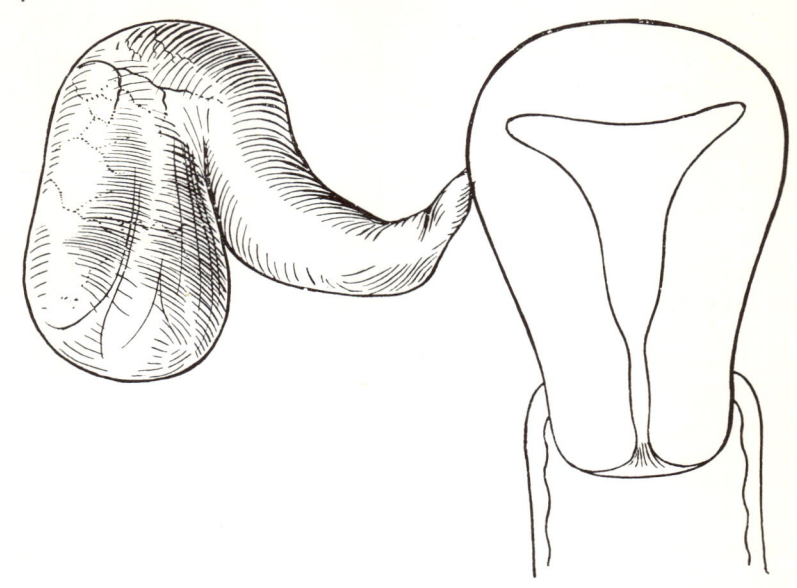

FIG. 36. Pyosalpinx. The right Fallopian tube is filled with pus. Since the ampulla is the most distensible part, it stretches considerably and the tube assumes this characteristic shape.

most distensible part, so that the dilated pus-filled tube or PYOSALPINX is typically the shape of a laboratory retort.

The contents are at first purulent, but in about four weeks in a favourable case the infection dies out, serous fluid replaces the pus, and the watery swelling remaining is called a HYDROSALPINX.

Acute suppurative salpingitis is an infection involving the whole tube, which is red and œdematous, frequently exuding pus from the abdominal ostium and causing pelvic peritonitis. Adhesions to neighbouring structures occur, notably the ovary, which may become involved in the suppuration to form a TUBO-OVARIAN ABSCESS. An acute infection may either subside completely, or may pass into a chronic stage. Adhesions to the uterus may cause painful retroversion, or backward displacement, of that organ.

Acute Salpingitis

Signs and Symptoms. The history is usually one of an acute cervical or uterine infection, e.g. gonorrhœa,

DISORDERS OF THE FALLOPIAN TUBES

septic abortion or puerperal infection. This provides the primary focus, which when it spreads to the tubes causes such constitutional signs as fever, anorexia and a rise in the white cell count. Pain in the lower abdomen, on both sides, is now a marked feature, and a vaginal examination by the surgeon will reveal acute local tenderness most marked on each side of the uterus. Pus may be found on the examining finger and a culture of this or from the cervix may reveal the causative organism.

The symptoms of acute salpingitis frequently follow the first menstrual period after an acute cervical or uterine infection. This, and subsequent periods, are likely to be excessive and prolonged unless the infection is rapidly cured.

Difficulties in diagnosis usually occur because of the natural disinclination of the patient to disclose that she has had a venereal infection, or a criminal abortion. The importance of failure to diagnose a case of acute appendicitis is obvious; it may lead to gangrene of the appendix and peritonitis. Every care is taken to exclude this condition on clinical evidence, but if this cannot be done with confidence it is best to perform a laparotomy, and if salpingitis is found, to close the abdomen.

Treatment of Acute Salpingitis

Once the diagnosis is made, the patient is put to bed comfortably supported with pillows. If a purulent vaginal discharge is present, precautions should be taken to prevent spread of infection to other patients. A swab is taken from the cervix for culture, and to discover the sensitivity of the organism to antibiotics, but treatment with wide-spectrum antibiotics is commenced immediately, and changed later if the sensitivities of the organism so dictate.

A four-hourly temperature, pulse and respiration chart is kept, and close watch maintained on her condition. The fluid output and intake is measured, and an intake of 3,000 ml. in twenty-four hours is aimed at. Frequent painful micturition would call for examination of a midstream specimen, and if sulphonamides are given the urine may be kept alkaline by giving potassium citrate. Pain is relieved by aspirin, codeine or pethidine, and heat to the lower abdomen is often prescribed.

Hot douches are not now often used in the treatment of salpingitis, but if ordered, six pints at a temperature rising gradually to 46° C. (115° F.) should be used, at very low pressure to avoid spreading infection upwards.

Chronic Salpingitis

Chronic inflammation of the Fallopian tube (with the exception of tuberculous salpingitis) is always preceded by an attack of acute salpingitis, although a history of such an attack is not invariably forthcoming. The ovaries may also be involved (salpingo-oöphoritis).

A patient with such a chronic inflammation usually complains of heavy menstrual loss, and has pain for a few days before the period begins. Backache is common, and so is pain during intercourse (dyspareunia). She may be anæmic from the excessive loss, and frequently complains of a muco-purulent vaginal discharge. On pelvic examination the uterus and appendages are tender, enlarged and fixed.

Treatment

Chronic salpingitis is a mixture of residual infection and fibrosis, together with adhesions to surrounding structures. Any residual infection should be treated by a prolonged course of antibiotic even though it is difficult or impossible to isolate the causative organisms at this late stage. Short-wave diathermy is of little or no value in curing any infection, although it may sometimes relieve symptoms such as backache. Frequently, however, the pain is due not to residual infection, but to adhesions, and surgery is the only effective treatment. Where a pyosalpinx or hydrosalpinx is present, the affected tube must be removed, and occasionally the ovary is so involved that it must also be sacrificed (salpingo-oöphorectomy). If the uterus is bound down by adhesions to the pouch of Douglas it should be freed (see p. 131). After operations of this sort, in which adhesions have had to be divided, intestinal obstruction may result from a loop of gut becoming adherent to a raw area. Vomiting and colicky pain occurring after about three days give rise to fears of this complication, and should be reported early to the surgeon. Measurements of the fluid taken and vomited should be kept, a specimen of the vomit

DISORDERS OF THE FALLOPIAN TUBES 87

is saved, and observation made on abdominal distension and whether flatus is being passed. The temperature remains low, and the pulse rate shows a progressive rise in a typical case. A Ryle's tube is passed transnasally into the stomach, and suction with a 50 ml. syringe made frequently enough to prevent vomiting. If intestinal contents can be withdrawn when no fluid is being taken by mouth, obstruction of some kind is certainly present. If it is of a mechanical nature, intravenous fluids are given in quantity sufficient to restore the fluid balance, and the patient is prepared for an operation to relieve the obstruction as soon as possible.

Tuberculous Salpingitis

Tuberculosis of the Fallopian tubes rarely presents in

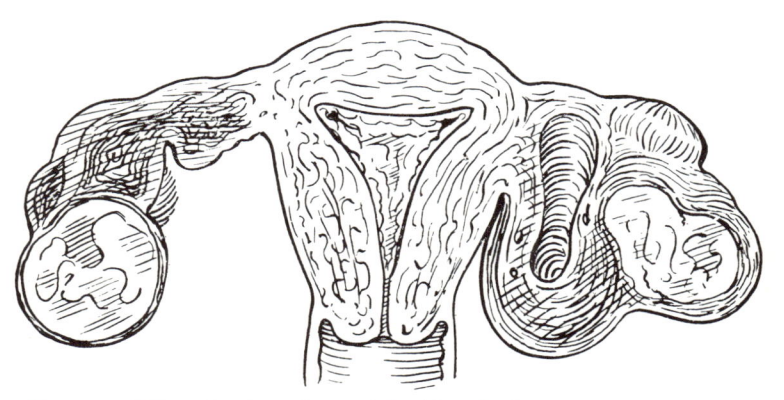

FIG. 37. Bilateral tuberculous salpingitis. Both Fallopian tubes are thickened by chronic inflammation. Section shows that the tubes are full of caseous material typical of tuberculosis.

an acute form. The patient is usually a young woman who has abdominal pain, worse before and during the periods, general debility, and, if married, may complain of infertility. In the early stages it is not uncommon for this disease to be revealed at laparotomy for what was thought to be recurrent appendicitis. In more advanced stages, bilateral pyosalpinx may occur with spread of the infection throughout the pelvis.

Surgery in such cases where adhesions are numerous is difficult, and apt to give rise to fæcal fistulæ. Skill and experience is needed to decide which patients will benefit from surgery, and what the scope of the operation should be. The usual sanatorium regime with rest, chemotherapy, fresh air and graduated exercise is of great importance to all patients.

NEW GROWTHS OF THE FALLOPIAN TUBE

It is unusual to meet a primary new growth of the Fallopian tube, and malignant disease affecting the tube has usually spread to it either from the ovary or the uterus. A growth beginning in the Fallopian tube is difficult to distinguish clinically from an ovarian new growth, and the treatment is the same, i.e. radical removal of the uterus and appendages.

ECTOPIC GESTATION

Fertilization of the ovum takes place within the Fallopian tube, which by peristalsis and ciliary action assists its progress to the uterine cavity, where normally it embeds itself in the upper part of the body of the uterus. In certain circumstances the fertilized ovum may attach itself somewhere outside the uterus and begin to grow. Such an extra-uterine pregnancy is called ECTOPIC GESTATION, and the majority of cases occur within the Fallopian tube. Very occasionally the ovary is the site of implantation. Even more rarely a tubal pregnancy may become detached from its origin and become secondarily implanted somewhere within the abdominal cavity (secondary abdominal pregnancy). Such a fœtus may grow to a fair size within the abdominal cavity, then die and undergo calcification, in which state it may be retained within the abdomen for many years. Such a stone baby, or LITHOPÆDION, is not likely to be encountered in this country, but may still be met where medical services are less easily available. In an exceptional case a secondary abdominal pregnancy has produced a live child, when the condition has been diagnosed in time for laparotomy to be performed, but almost invariably an ectopic gestation results at an early stage in the death of the fœtus, and the resulting intraperitoneal hæmorrhage may threaten the life of the patient.

DISORDERS OF THE FALLOPIAN TUBES

Many causes have been suggested for ectopic pregnancy. A history of previous inflammation in the tubes is sometimes forthcoming, and adhesions are thought to delay the onward passage of the ovum. Sometimes at operation ectopic gestation may be seen in a Fallopian tube, while the presence of a corpus luteum in the opposite ovary indicates that the ovum had to traverse the peritoneal cavity before entering the Fallopian tube. Sometimes no abnormality can be detected, and it is then supposed that the ovum has an unduly tendency to early implantation.

TUBAL PREGNANCY

Once implantation has occurred in the tube, the sequence of events normally associated with pregnancy follows. The corpus luteum remains and grows, producing progesterone which increases the thickness of the endometrium and ensures that it is not shed, so that the patient misses a period. The tube is not, however, able to nourish the ovum for more than a few weeks, and either bleeding

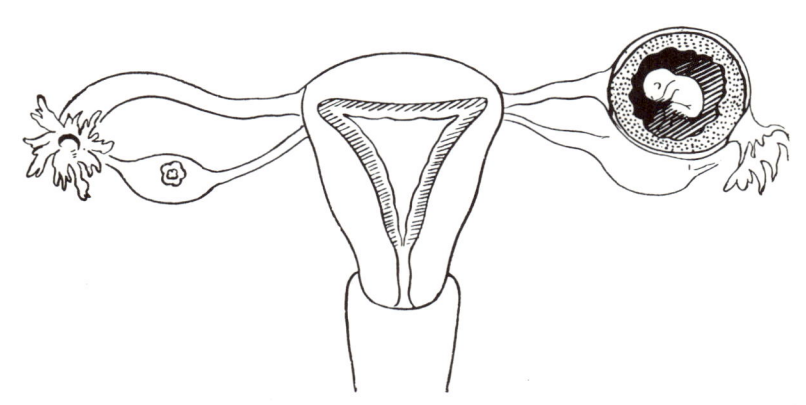

FIG. 38. Diagram of tubal (ectopic) gestation. The left tube is the site of pregnancy, and a corpus luteum is shown in the right ovary. The endometrium in the uterus shows the decidual reaction characteristic of pregnancy.

detaches the ovum, which may be ejected into the peritoneal cavity through the fimbriated end, or the wall of the tube is eroded and ruptures, often with intraperitoneal bleeding on a dangerous scale. These two types of a case present a rather different clinical picture and will be described separately.

If the ovum is detached from the tube by bleeding it dies, and may either remain in the tube as a TUBAL MOLE, or pass into the peritoneal cavity—TUBAL ABORTION. The patient's chief complaint is of pain, severe, usually colicky, and often causing nausea and fainting. On questioning she may give a history of a missed period, and may believe herself pregnant, having noticed morning sickness and breast changes, but the bleeding may come too soon for such a history to be obtained. Within a day of the death of the ovum, the decidua in the uterus is cast off, and vaginal bleeding follows. The nurse must remember that the amount lost per vaginam is not the only loss; blood clot in some quantity is accumulating in and around the tube.

A patient in whom ectopic gestation has been diagnosed should always be admitted to hospital immediately, because skilled observation is essential. Urgent operation is required for the removal of an ectopic pregnancy, though surgery may be avoided in some patients with tubal mole or abortion. Even though operation is not at once urgent in many cases of tubal mole or abortion, it may become so, and the patient needs to be under skilled observation. Salpingectomy, or removal of the affected tube, will have to be performed.

TUBAL RUPTURE
(RUPTURED ECTOPIC GESTATION)

If the Fallopian tube is eroded by the ectopic gestation, what happens is decided by the position of the ovum within the tube. If it is attached to the upper part of the tube, rupture will be into the peritoneal cavity, and may be accompanied by diffuse and severe intra-abdominal bleeding. Should it be attached to the lowest part of the tube, it will rupture between the two layers of the broad ligament, which will be forced apart by the bleeding to form a BROAD LIGAMENT HÆMATOMA.

In either case, the dominating feature of the clinical picture is the signs of internal bleeding described on p. 45. Sudden and severe abdominal pain, often causing fainting, is felt at the moment of rupture, and the signs of concealed bleeding become progressively more obvious. The patient

DISORDERS OF THE FALLOPIAN TUBES

is blanched and sweating, with a low temperature and blood pressure, and a pulse rising in rate and diminishing in volume. The lower abdomen may be tender and rigid, and some distension may be seen. The story of a missed period, and early signs of activity in the breasts are of assistance if present in diagnosing ruptured tubal gestation from other acute abdominal emergencies.

Operation is urgent, and very little preparation is needed. The patient is given a pre-operative injection such as atropine 0·6 mgm. and morphine 10 mgm. and dressed for the theatre. The operation area must be shaved, but this might be painful if the abdomen is distended and tender, and it may well be done in the anæsthetic room when the patient is unconscious. The bladder must be emptied by catheter, and this should also be done in the theatre.

However serious the patient's condition appears to be, the results of operation are excellent. The abdomen is opened and the ruptured tube removed, the ovary being conserved if possible. Blood clot is removed, and the wound sutured. Transfusion has meanwhile been begun, the head of the table is lowered, and the patient remains on the table until her condition is good enough for her to return to the ward. A remarkable improvement immediately follows suturing of the bleeding vessel.

The post-operative period is usually uneventful. Vaginal bleeding will begin 12 to 24 hours after the death of the ovum, so a sterile pad is applied and regular perineal toilet undertaken. The absorption of blood from anywhere within the body causes a little fever, as the nurse will remember in connection with fractures, or subarachnoid hæmorrhage, and this patient will show a similar reaction. A temperature of 37·2° to 37·8° C. (99° to 100° F.) is to be expected during the first week, and does not necessarily mean that any complication will occur.

This operation is no bar to a future pregnancy and many patients subsequently enjoy a normal gestation. It is also true that in 5% of these patients an ectopic pregnancy will occur in the remaining Fallopian tube.

CHAPTER 7
DISORDERS OF THE UTERUS

Anatomy and Physiology

The uterus is 7·5 to 9 cm. (3 to 3½ in.) long, 5 to 6 cm. (2 to 2½ in.) wide in its upper part and 2·5 cm. (1 in.) thick, its bulk being due to its muscular middle coat. Its parts are named as follows:—

The FUNDUS is the part above the opening of the Fallopian tubes into the uterine cavity.

The BODY is the middle main portion.

The CERVIX is the lowest part, which projects into the vagina.

The cervical canal opens into the uterine cavity at the INTERNAL OS, and its vaginal orifice is the EXTERNAL OS.

The lining of the uterus is the ENDOMETRIUM, which is shed monthly at menstruation, and the muscle layer is the MYOMETRIUM.

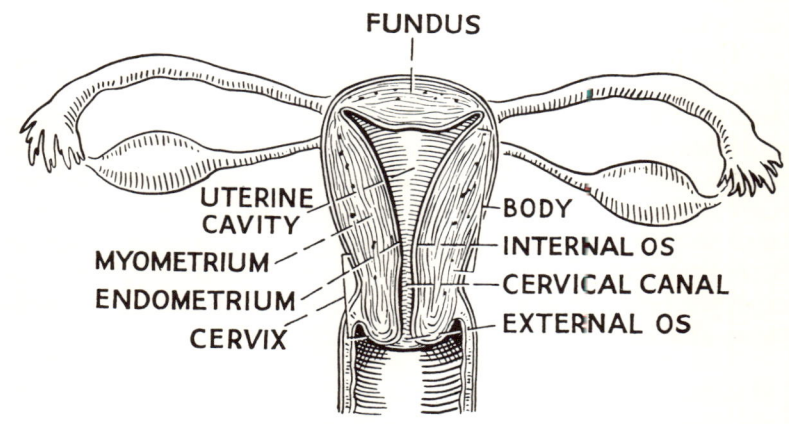

FIG. 39. Diagrammatic section through the uterus.

The body is bent forwards upon the cervix at the level of the internal os, and the whole uterus leans forward over the bladder, so that its normal position is one of ANTEFLEXION and ANTEVERSION. Peritoneum is

DISORDERS OF THE UTERUS

reflected from the bladder over the front of the uterus, over the fundus and down the posterior aspect of the uterus onto the posterior vaginal fornix whence it is reflected onto the anterior aspect of the rectum. The part lying between the uterus and the front of the rectum being the POUCH OF DOUGLAS. The uterine artery runs along the lower edge of the broad ligament, and its branches pursue a tortuous course which enables the uterus to expand in pregnancy without stretching its vessels.

Supports of the Uterus. Since much gynæcological surgery is concerned with correcting descent of the uterus and its neighbouring structures, it is important to realize what normally keeps the uterus in position. There are three main factors:—

(1) The muscles of the pelvic floor, principally the levator ani, in so far as these muscles support the pelvic viscera in general. The pelvic floor slopes downwards

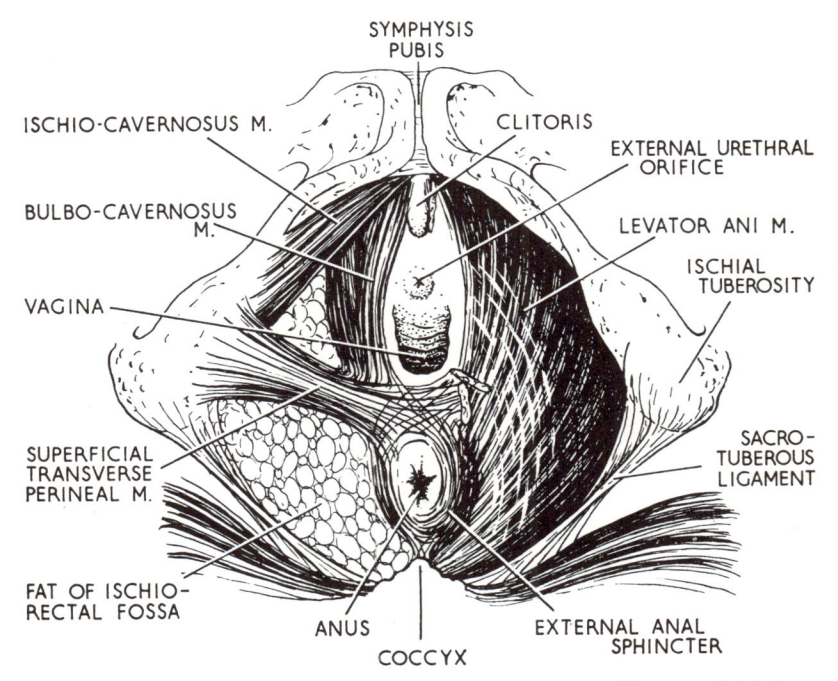

FIG. 40. The structure of the pelvic floor, seen from below. The superficial tissue have been removed from the right hand side to show the most important muscle, levator ani.

and forwards, and is traversed in the mid-line by the urethra, vagina and rectum. While these muscles are intact and of good tone, descent or prolapse of the pelvic contents is unlikely.

(2) The ligaments of the uterus help to retain it in position. They are of unequal importance in this respect. A. The TRANSVERSE, or CARDINAL or MACKENRODT'S ligaments pass from the cervix and vagina to the side wall of the pelvis and have the greatest supporting value. B. The UTERO-SACRAL ligaments which are part of the transverse ligaments run backwards from the cervix to the sacrum. C. The ROUND LIGAMENTS are bands attached to the uterus in front of the Fallopian tubes which run forwards into the inguinal canals and so into the labia majora. These are unimportant as supports. D. The BROAD LIGAMENT has already been described in connection with the Fallopian tubes,

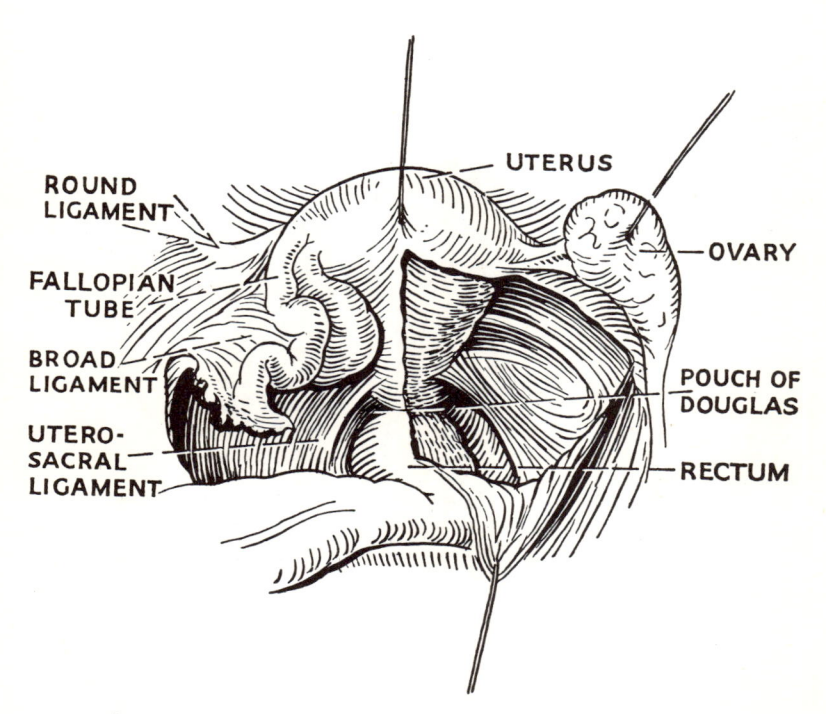

FIG. 41. The uterus and its appendages; posterior aspect.

DISORDERS OF THE UTERUS

This fold of peritoneum is of great anatomical importance, but is not a means of support.

The uterine conditions for which medical advice may be sought can be summarized as follows:—

(1) Congenital abnormalities.
(2) Infections. Information on these will be found in the chapter on venereal disease, and on infection following childbirth
(3) Disorders of menstruation.
(4) New growths, innocent and malignant.
(5) Prolapse of the uterus and its related structures.

Congenital Abnormalities

The Fallopian tubes, uterus and vagina are formed within the female fetus from a pair of primitive structures, the Müllerian ducts. These fuse in the midline, so that though the Fallopian tubes are paired the uterus and vagina are single. Failure of fusion may occur, and in extreme cases the uterus, cervix and vagina are double. It is not uncommon for the uterus to remain rudimentary and undeveloped, and sometimes the vagina is partly or completely absent.

Some of these abnormalities give rise to few symptoms, and pregnancy and delivery may take place without incident. Some of them, such as uterus subseptus, illustrated here, are amenable to surgery if they cause repeated abortion, as they sometimes do.

Congenital absence of the vagina can also sometimes be

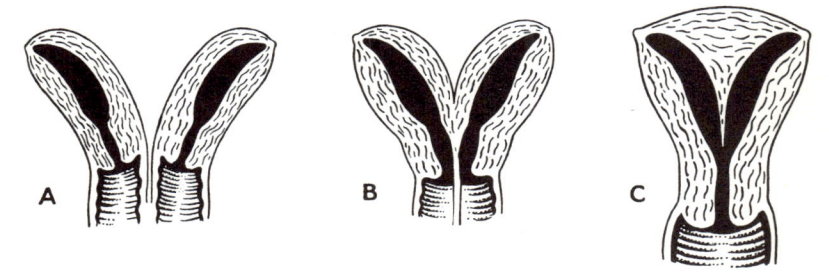

FIG. 42. Some congenital abnormalities of the uterus and vagina.
A. Uterus and vagina may be double (uterus didelphys).
B. Less complete forms of duplication are found.
C. The uterine cavity may be partially divided by a septum (uterus subseptus).

remedied by surgery, though since a normal uterus is rarely present in such cases the patient is only occasionally made capable of bearing children. A space is made between the rectum and the urethra, and the surgeon lines this cavity with skin by means of grafts applied on a mould. This must be kept in place for three months to secure a satisfactory result.

Disorders of Menstruation

Normal menstruation occurs every twenty-four to thirty days, and lasts for three to seven days, the amount lost being 60 to 180 ml. Every woman tends to keep to the same pattern throughout the reproductive period of her life. Pain of a disabling nature should be absent, but mild discomfort before and during menstruation is usual. These terms are used in connection with menstrual symptoms.

AMENORRHŒA means absence of menstruation.

OLIGOMENORRHŒA is scanty and HYPOMENORRHŒA is infrequent menstruation.

EPI- or POLYMENORRHŒA indicates that the periods occur at shorter intervals than usual.

MENORRHAGIA means that the loss is heavier than usual.

DYSMENORRHŒA is painful menstruation.

METRORRHAGIA is the term used for irregular genital bleeding. Though not menstrual in origin, patients are not always able to distinguish this, and it is convenient to discuss it here.

AMENORRHŒA is normal before ovarian activity begins at puberty, after it has ceased at the menopause, during pregnancy, and for some months after delivery. PRIMARY amenorrhœa means that menstruation has never occurred, SECONDARY amenorrhœa that the periods, previously present, have ceased. A woman during the reproductive period who complains of amenorrhœa should be examined for signs of pregnancy. Other causes may be grouped under the following headings:—

(1) **Endocrine.** The ovaries may be underactive; pituitary, suprarenal or thyroid disorders may be present. Diabetes is another cause of amenorrhœa.

DISORDERS OF THE UTERUS

(2) Nervous. A change of occupation or environment often causes suppression of the periods for a month or two, especially in young girls. Fear of or desire for pregnancy, sudden shocks or anxiety are other causes. The influence of the central nervous system on menstruation is powerful if not well understood.

(3) Constitutional. Severe debilitating diseases such

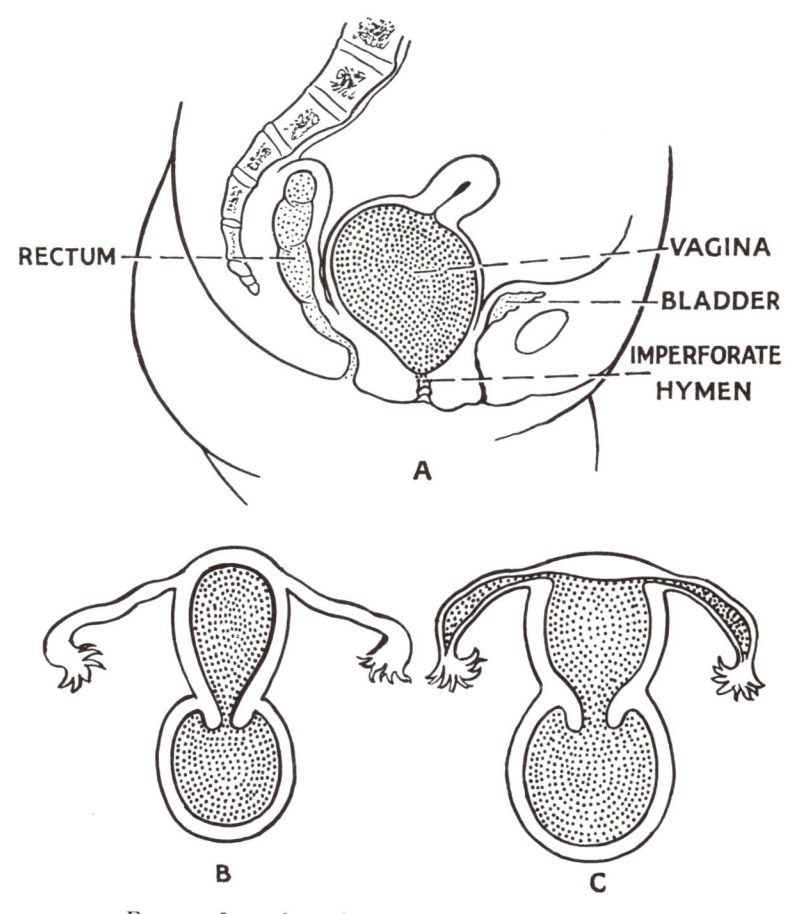

Fig. 43. Imperforate hymen causing cryptomenorrhœa.
A. Hæmatocolpos. The menstrual flow is retained in the vagina, which becomes progressively distended.
B. In long-standing cases the uterine cavity may also become filled with blood—hæmatometra.
C. In time the Fallopian tubes become similarly distended—hæmatosalpynx. Cases of such severity are uncommon.

as tuberculosis and profound anæmia may interrupt the periods. So may specific fevers.

(4) **Local.** After hysterectomy, bilateral oöphorectomy or exposure to full doses of radiation, menstruation cannot return.

(5) A congenital abnormality that causes what is apparently primary amenorrhœa is IMPERFORATE HYMEN. The vaginal orifice is closed by an intact membrane, so that the menstrual fluid is retained in the vagina, a condition called HÆMATOCOLPOS. If left long untreated the uterus and tubes may become distended with blood, but this is unusual. The condition is simply cured by incision of the hymen in most cases.

Treatment. If the condition is secondary to some local or general condition, this must of course be treated. In girls who have never menstruated, a course of hormone treatment may be successful in producing uterine bleeding, but not necessarily ovulation. OLIGOMENORRHŒA and HYPOMENORRHŒA usually occur together; the interval between the periods is long and the loss slight. Its causes and treatment are similar to amenorrhœa of other than physiological cases. It is sometimes associated with underdevelopment of the genitalia or an infantile type of ovary, and is probably secondary to anterior pituitary deficiency. Chromosome studies and estimation of the amount of follicle stimulating hormone will usually reveal the cause in those patients who are not suffering from obvious disease.

Epimenorrhœa

This occurs commonly when menstruation starts or finishes, e.g. at puberty or the menopause. It is also seen after pregnancy when menstruation is being re-established, or at the menopause, and sometimes fibroids (*q.v.*) cause epimenorrhœa. No treatment is indicated except in the presence of fibroids, or when severe loss occurs at the menopause.

MENORRHAGIA is important because if it is long continued it will lead to anæmia. It is a symptom, not a disease, and its cause must be sought. Common causes

DISORDERS OF THE UTERUS

are chronic pelvic infection, fibromyomata of the uterus and retroversion of the uterus, and the treatment of the cause will cure the heavy loss.

Another important group of cases is hormonal in origin, and of these METROPATHIA HÆMORRHAGICA is the one of the more common. It is caused by the unopposed action of an excess amount of œstrogen from the ovary, and is recognized by the patient having prolonged phases of amenorrhœa, which are followed by continuous heavy bleeding for many days. This excessive œstrogen production inhibits ovulation, as a result of which such patients are sterile. Since there is no ovulation, no corpus luteum is produced, and the endometrium never shows those changes associated with progesterone secretion, so that it does not progress beyond the proliferative stage.

Although the condition is due to œstrogen excess, progesterone deficiency is present and treatment with progesterone is often successful temporarily, and sometimes in the long term. Curettage of the uterus may prove beneficial temporarily and must be performed to establish a diagnosis but in older women hysterectomy has to be

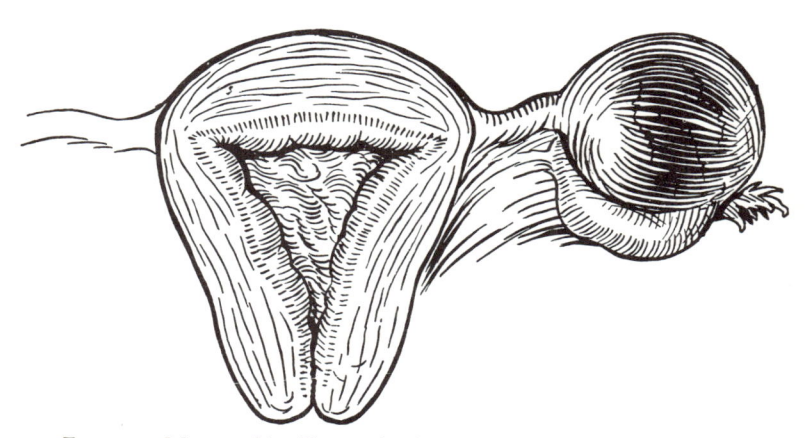

FIG. 44. Metropathia Hæmorrhagica. The myometrium is hypertrophied and the endometrium thickened. The left ovary contains a cyst.

considered. General measures to raise the hæmoglobin level are always necessary, and transfusion is often required, especially if operation is being considered.

Young women usually respond satisfactorily to progesterone by mouth.

Metrorrhagia

This term is often used rather vaguely in speaking of irregular bleeding, and the important thing for the nurse to bear constantly in mind about this symptom is that it is one of the early signs of cancer of the uterus. Any patient complaining of it during or after the reproductive period should be examined by a gynæcologist with a view to excluding the possibility of malignant disease. A digital and speculum examination of the cervix together with cervical and vaginal smears for cytological examination are always necessary and in any case of doubt, where the cervix appears normal, the uterus is curetted. Nurses are not infrequently consulted by friends and acquaintances about such symptoms, and they should most strongly urge immediate medical examination, since the prospect of a cure of a carcinoma of cervix is said to decrease by 2% with every week that passes from the onset of symptoms.

Vaginal bleeding may be caused by a polypus projecting from the uterus into the vagina, especially a submucous fibroid polypus (p. 105), by incomplete evacuation of the uterus after an abortion; or following cessation of a course of an œstrogen like stilbœstrol. Metrorrhagia should never be dismissed without a full and thorough examination, if necessary under an anæsthetic.

Pain during menstruation is termed DYSMENORRHŒA. It is a symptom, not a disease, and it must be recognized at once that there are few women who have never experienced any discomfort at menstruation. A feeling of abdominal distension commonly precedes the period and some backache and tenderness in the lower abdomen may be felt. Symptoms of water retention, such as swelling of the ankles, are often noted which disperses as menstruation begins, with a noticeable polyuria. Tenderness may be felt in the breasts, mental irritability or an ill-defined sense of tension and unease as the period approaches. These symptoms are mainly physiological and not disabling. Sometimes, however, pain is severe enough to interfere with the patient's normal life and make her seek medical advice. The number of patients referred to

DISORDERS OF THE UTERUS

gynæcological clinics with dysmenorrhœa has fallen dramatically. This may be because there is a variety of proprietary preparations available for relief of pain, but probably also reflects a more matter of fact attitude to menstruation among girls and the desirability of holding a desirable post.

Dysmenorrhœa can be discussed under two headings:

(a) Primary or Spasmodic Dysmenorrhœa

This term covers the majority of cases. Typically the patient is a girl in her teens, who developed her troubles a few years after puberty. At the onset of the period and for a few hours afterwards she experiences pain low in the abdomen, usually at the front, but sometimes in the back. It is colicky in nature, and sometimes excruciatingly severe, causing nausea, vomiting and fainting. It rarely lasts longer than the first day, and then disappears and does not return. She is most likely to be a sedentary worker, often introspective, but it may occur in every type of woman. If she marries and has children the condition almost always cures itself, but even without children it is unusual for it to persist throughout the reproductive period; it begins to decline in severity during the thirties.

The cause of the pain is unknown, but many theories have been advanced, of which the following are the most popular.

(1) **Obstructive.** The cervical canal is thought to be small and rigid, so that pain is experienced during the expulsion of the menstrual products. Certainly women with a small infantile type of uterus often experience dysmenorrhœa.

(2) **Muscular Imbalance.** The cervix should relax when the body of the uterus contracts to expel the flow, and failure to do so may cause pain.

(3) **Endocrine Dysharmony.** A lack of balance between œstrogen and progesterone has been suggested.

(4) **Nervous Origin.** No doubt some cases are made worse by psychological factors; the terms used of menstruation in some classes of society indicate this clearly. Being " unwell " or " poorly " has a strong suggestion of invalidism. This kind of attitude should be deprecated, and the nurse in her capacity as health teacher may help.

(5) **Ischæmia.** Pain may be caused by spasm of the

vessels, as it is in the legs when vascular disorders reduce the blood supply. The type of uterus most likely to suffer from ischæmia is the underdeveloped one. Some of these patients have a demonstrably low pain threshold, and may be disabled by pain that another woman might class as discomfort. However, the prospect of a regular return of severe pain every twenty-eight days would be daunting even to the best-adjusted temperament, and sympathetic help should be given.

Treatment. First and foremost the patient must be convinced that the pain does not indicate any disease although those who suffer from incapacitating pain should be examined by a doctor. If the patient is an indoor worker with poor circulation much can be done on general lines. She is told that exercise will benefit the condition, and if possible it should be outdoors in the company of young people. The physiotherapist may teach her exercises to improve her abdominal and pelvic muscles. She is told that constipation will make the pain worse and a simple saline aperient may be prescribed before the period is due. This will also help in dispersing the fluid retention that causes the swelling of the ankles. Hot bottles at the onset of the period are comforting and an analgesic of the aspirin or codeine type should be given for use when the period begins. She is advised not to go to bed if it can be avoided.

It is useless to tell a young girl that she will be better after having had a baby, but if she is married she may be informed of the fact. Many women will improve with a better routine like the one described, but a number of cases remain in which further measures are needed.

Spasmodic dysmenorrhœa indicates that ovulation has occurred, and patients can be reassured concerning this vital function and also that suppression of ovulation will nearly always relieve the pain. This is usually achieved by giving small doses of œstrogen (stilbœstrol 1 mgm. daily) or progesterone (nor-ethisterone 5 mgm. daily) for twenty-one days, starting on the fifth day of the menstrual cycle. This treatment is usually continued for six months, after which relief continues for an indefinite period. The most convenient method of suppressing ovulation is by the use of the contraceptive pill, some types of which have been used in the above form for more than 30 years.

DISORDERS OF THE UTERUS

Dilatation of the cervix is also practised. Under a general anæsthetic the cervix is dilated up to No. 14 Hegar, and a glass rod may be left in for twenty-four hours. Following this 25% of patients will be cured, 50% will be improved, and the remainder in six months' time may again be in pain. This operation, however, predisposes to abortion in the middle of subsequent pregnancies and is only performed in the most severe cases when all else has failed.

In rare instances, where all measures conscientiously carried out have failed, some surgeons used to consider the operation of sympathetic denervation of the uterus. Briefly, the operation consists in cutting, by an abdominal approach, all the sensory nerves to the uterus.

(b) Secondary Dysmenorrhœa

Secondary or congestive dysmenorrhœa. Patients with this symptom may be of any age, and menstruation is normal when first established, pain only arising later. A young woman with primary dysmenorrhœa usually has no other complaints, but since secondary dysmenorrhœa, as its name implies, is produced by some other conditions, the patient usually shows other symptoms too.

The pain usually begins two or three days before the onset of bleeding, sometimes as long as a week before. It is a heavy, dragging ache, felt throughout the pelvis, and often spreading into the back and the inner aspects of the thighs. Once bleeding is well established, the pain gradually disappears, but the loss is often abnormally heavy (menorrhagia) and lasts longer than usual. Often the cycle is shortened (epimenorrhœa) so that the interval between the periods is reduced. The patient is thus in the depressing state of spending most of the time menstruating, or suffering from pain ahead of the next period. If this condition persists for any length of time, anæmia will result from the frequent heavy periods.

Secondary dysmenorrhœa is a symptom, and the cause must be sought. It is sometimes a complaint of women in whom no pelvic abnormality is found, and the congestion may be due to emotional causes, such as a sex life that involves more stimulation than satisfaction. The commonest cause is chronic salpingitis, especially if there are pelvic adhesions causing fixed retroversion of the uterus. The treatment is that of the cause, and is described in chapter 6. Anæmia must be corrected if present.

NEW GROWTHS OF THE UTERUS
A. BENIGN

I. Fibromyomata (Fibroids)

These tumours are the commonest new growth of the uterus being composed of plain muscle and fibrous tissue. They are practically confined to the uterus, in which they may occur in great numbers, varying in size from minute seedling growths to tumours weighing several pounds. They do not arise before puberty or after the menopause, and are usually seen in women of thirty to fifty years who have not borne children. Though common in Europeans, they are commoner still in negroid women.

The association between infertility and fibroids is well marked, and it has been held that one causes the other, though removal of a fibroid will not necessarily cure the infertility. Many of these patients have cystic ovaries and a thickened endometrium suggestive of excessive œstrogen

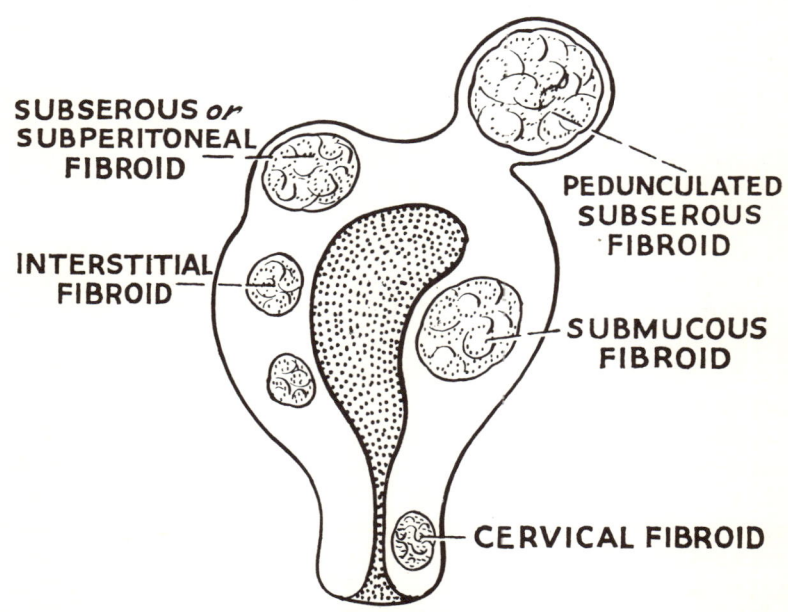

FIG. 45. Types of uterine fibroid.

production, and possibly this upset of hormone balance causes both the infertility and the fibroids.

The tumours are solid and spherical with a well-marked capsule, affect the body of the uterus (95%) more often than the cervix (5%), and may occupy any position in the uterine wall. The symptoms they cause vary with their position, and the following types are described:

(1) **Submucous Fibroids.** These lie immediately under the endometrium and project into the uterine cavity, the shape of which they may grossly distort. Sometimes such a tumour may develop a pedicle, and project into the endometrial cavity as a fibroid polyp; rarely a fibroid polyp is extruded through the cervix to project into the vagina. These tumours distort the endometrial cavity and cause menorrhagia.

(2) **Interstitial Fibroids.** These occur in the uterine muscle, and all fibroids are first interstitial in type, and either pass inwards to become submucous or outwards, when they are included in the next class. They rarely cause symptoms.

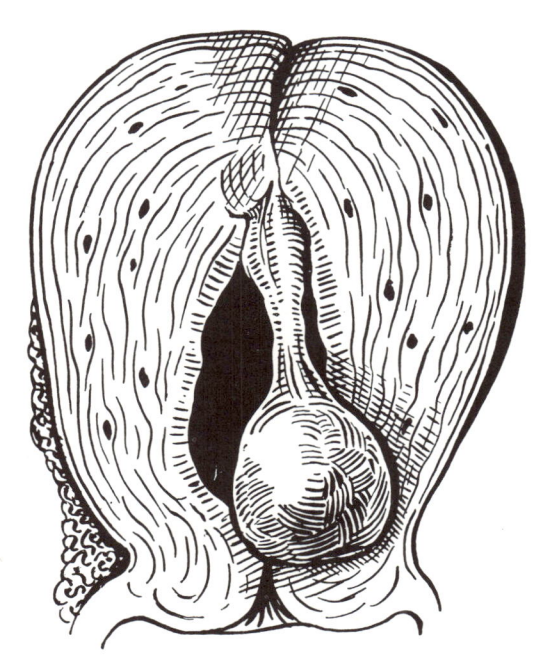

Fig. 46. Fibroid polypus of the uterus.

(3) **Subserous or Subperitoneal Fibroids.** These grow outwards into the peritoneal cavity. They are frequently multiple, and may grow to a large size when they cause pressure symptoms, especially disturbances of micturition.

(4) **Cervical Fibroids.** These are usually small but if they grow to a size of several centimetres in diameter may cause obstructed labour.

Signs and Symptoms

(1) **Menorrhagia.** Prolonged and excessive menstrual loss is the commonest symptom of interstitial and submucous fibroids, and is due partly to the thickened endometrium and partly to the increase in size of the uterine cavity which they cause. It may give rise to a profound anæmia.

(2) **Pressure Symptoms.** These are especially frequent with subserous fibroids, which because of their situation tend to be fixed in the pelvis. FREQUENCY OF MICTURITION occurs because the bladder has little

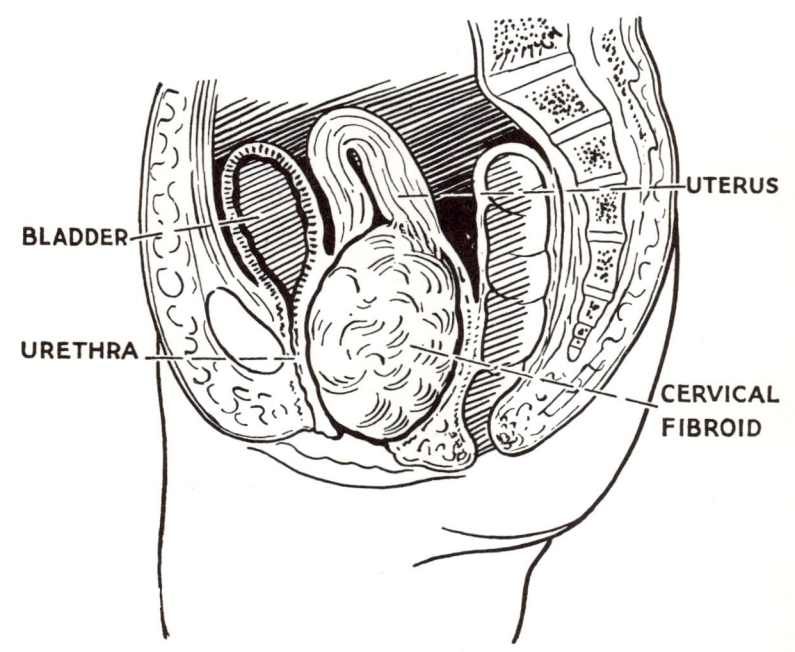

FIG. 47. A cervical fibroid causing retention of urine by stretching the urethra and pressing on it.

room to expand, and retention of urine may occur later. HÆMORRHOIDS and VARICOSE VEINS are due to pressure on the pelvic veins.

(3) **Abdominal swelling** only occurs with big subperitoneal and multiple interstitial fibroids projecting into the abdominal cavity. A lump will be felt in the abdomen.

(4) **Infertility.** Even though the patient's childlessness is perhaps not directly caused by fibroids, it may bring her to her doctor for advice, and lead to the discovery of the growth.

Signs and symptoms also arise in connection with the complications to which fibroids are liable, and which are given below.

COMPLICATIONS

Degeneration. All fibroids atrophy after the menopause, but a variety of changes may take place in the growths before this. Clinically one of the most important is RED DEGENERATION. This is a peculiar type of necrosis of a fibroid, sometimes seen during pregnancy, and causing pyrexia, abdominal pain, constitutional upset and vomiting. The treatment during pregnancy is conservative. MALIGNANT degeneration can give rise to a sarcoma of uterus, but it is not a common occurrence, being seen in less than 0.5% of all fibroids. Other degenerations can occur, the commonest of which is hyaline. Here the substance of the tumour is replaced by a clear glassy material, in which calcium salts may later be deposited to form a womb-stone.

INFECTION of a fibroid is only likely if a submucous fibroid has been extruded through the cervix as a polypus. It is accompanied by bleeding and an offensive vaginal discharge.

Treatment of Fibromyomata

Several factors have to be assessed in deciding on the appropriate treatment. The size and number of the tumours, the severity of the symptoms, the age of the patient and her view on subsequent childbearing must all be considered. What would be appropriate treatment for a woman of forty-five with multiple tumours and menorrhagia would be unsuitable for a woman of thirty anxious to have a baby. The methods available may be summarized as follows:—

(1) **Expectant.** A woman nearing the menopause whose symptoms are not severe and who is unwilling to undergo operation should be treated conservatively, because these mild symptoms will be relieved when the periods cease at the menopause, and afterwards the fibroids will get smaller. Iron may be given to treat mild anæmia.

(2) **Operation.** This is the most widely used method of treatment. If the patient desires children and the growths

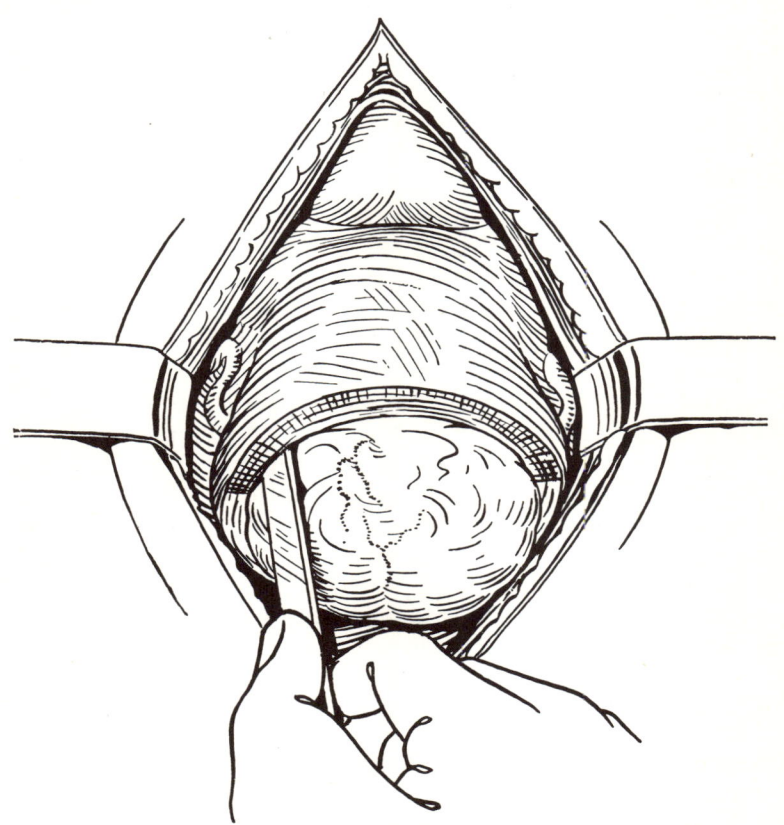

FIG. 48. Myomectomy. A large fibroid is being shelled out of the fundus of the uterus.

are amenable to excision, MYOMECTOMY or removal of the fibroid from the uterus may be undertaken. The uterus is exposed by an abdominal incision, and the fibroids shelled out; sometimes several can be removed through a single opening in the uterus. Hæmorrhage may occur after this operation, and the nurse must keep a record of the pulse at frequent intervals during the first few hours. Myomectomy is attractive in theory, but not always applicable in practice, especially if the tumours are numerous or situated near the Fallopian tubes.

HYSTERECTOMY is the operation of choice if the fibroids are very numerous or the patient is over forty. There is a general belief to-day that total hysterectomy is the operation of choice, since it eliminates the risk of subsequent carcinoma of cervix and any other disease of the cervical stump. If there is any prolapse present as well, the uterus can be removed by vaginal hysterectomy, and the prolapse repaired at the same time. This vaginal operation is only feasible for small fibroids. If the fibroid projects into the vagina as a polyp, it may be twisted off with a pair of ring forceps, or its pedicle may be cut with scissors. Little bleeding should occur if the pedicle is tied with a transfixing ligature.

II. Endometriomata

Chocolate cyst formation in connection with the ovaries has already been discussed, and the uterus is commonly affected by a similar condition. Tumours may appear in the uterine wall, and if the process is extensive hysterectomy will be required.

B. MALIGNANT NEW GROWTHS OF THE UTERUS

The uterus is second only to the breast as a site of malignant disease in women. 67% of these growths arise in the cervix as squamous cell carcinomata whilst 33% are adenocarcinomata arising from the body of the uterus. These two growths differ markedly in their pathology, spread, symptomatology, prognosis, and the type of patient who suffers from them.

Carcinoma of the cervix occurs almost always in women who have borne children (93%), the greatest number of patients are between forty-five and fifty-five, while it is not uncommon in women under forty. Since malignant disease tends in any situation to run a more rapid course in younger people, it is not surprising that the prognosis is worse than in carcinoma of the body of the uterus. Carcinoma of the body arises in an older age group (fifty-five to seventy) of which 80% have borne children.

Cancer arises in the cervix at the margin of the external os where it remains confined to it for some little time, then it begins to penetrate into neighbouring tissues. It extends outwards towards the pelvic wall, downwards into the vagina, backwards to the rectum and forward into the bladder. Lymphatic spread occurs quite early into the pelvic glands and thence to the glands of the lumbar region.

CARCINOMA OF THE CERVIX

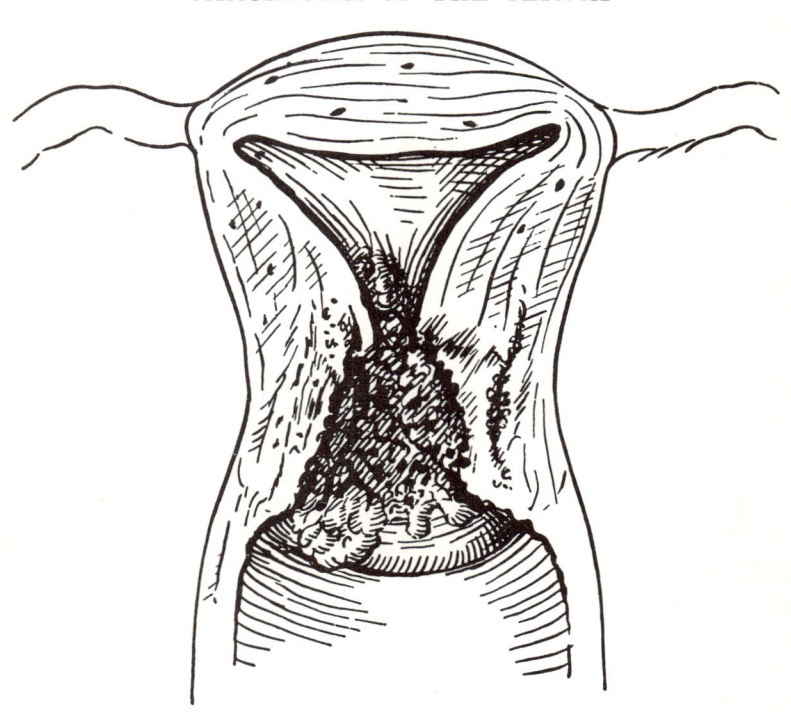

FIG. 49. Carcinoma of cervix. The growth is destroying the cervical tissue and spreading into the vault of the vagina.

Spread by the blood stream to bones or lungs is unusual, so that in far advanced cases the malignant process may not extend beyond the pelvis. It is a sad fact that more cases of extensive disease than early ones are seen, with corresponding decrease in the chances of cure. Everyone who

DISORDERS OF THE UTERUS

is in a position to induce such patients to seek expert advice early should do so, and nurses may play an important part here.

Signs and Symptoms

The patient is likely to be a woman of forty-five who has had at least one child and perhaps a history of chronic inflammation of the cervix following her last delivery. She first notices a little irregular vaginal bleeding, which she may attribute to the change of life. It is due to ulceration

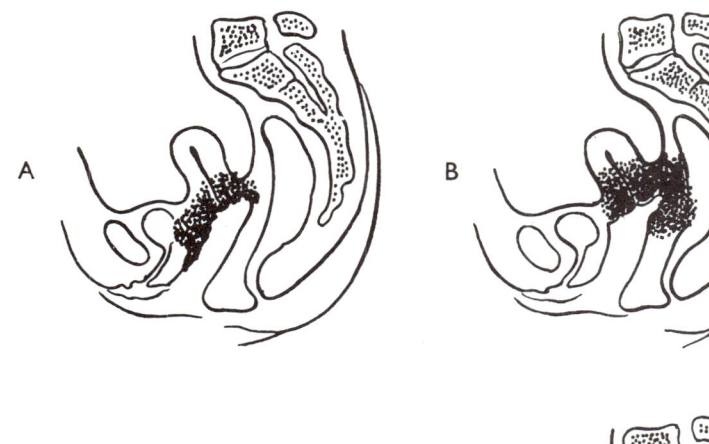

Fig. 50. Carcinoma of cervix, showing some methods of spread.
 A. The growth extends forward into the bladder.
 B. The pouch of Douglas and the anterior wall of the rectum are invaded.
 C. The vagina is extensively infiltrated and metastases may appear in the vulva.

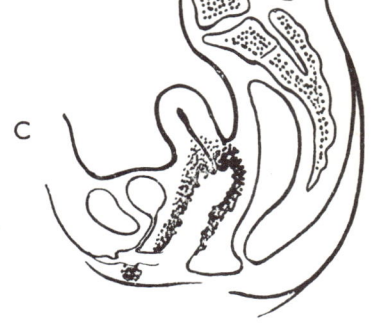

of the surface of the growth, and becomes heavier and more prolonged as time passes. Post coital bleeding, a bleeding after intercourse is one of the earliest and most important symptoms. The appearance of an offensive discharge indicates infection of the necrotic surface of the tumour. She becomes easily fatigued and pale as anæmia develops. It is most important to emphasize that pain is a symptom of advanced disease. While the growth is confined to the cervix there is no pain. Pain only occurs when the growth has spread to surrounding organs. Further symptoms depend on the direction of spread. If the bladder is involved, frequency of micturition and later hæmaturia and pain appear, and if the growth perforates the bladder to form a vesico-vaginal fistula, incontinence of urine follows. Recto-vaginal fistula and incontinence of fæces may result from backward spread, and extension beneath the broad ligament may involve the ureters. Death from ureteric obstruction occurs in over 50% of cases.

Diagnosis

As already indicated, the early diagnosis of cancer of the cervix is of paramount importance. The history may be suggestive, and physical examination will confirm the diagnosis. The cervix is irregular, hard, ulcerated, and bleeds easily when touched. A biopsy will confirm the presence of cancer.

Very early in the disease, however, the cervix may appear normal, but if a cancer is present it will be shedding malignant cells from its surface. These will be present in the cervical mucus and in the vagina, and they can be recognized by a cytologist when they are placed on a glass slide and stained by Papanicolau's method.

Cytology

Exfoliative cytology or the examination of cells which are continuously being shed from the cervix or vagina, is now an important part of any gynæcological examination.

The importance of the Smear or Papanicolau's test in the prevention of carcinoma of the cervix cannot be too strongly emphasized. Cancer of the cervix does not suddenly occur. Many years (up to 15 or 20 years) before the actual cancer develops there are changes in the squamous epithelium of the cervix which can be recognized by the smear test. Patients with such suspicious smears may then be admitted to hospital for cone biopsy of the cervix which will disclose the accurate histological condition. Basal cell hyperplasia and carcinoma in situ both of which may progress to actual cancer can be recognized by the smear test and if appropriate treatment is instituted the development of cancer of the cervix can be avoided.

Cytology is also used to assess the hormone levels because the cells of the vagina reflect the level of both œstrogen and progesterone. The presence of ovulation can also be determined.

Mucus is taken from both the cervix and the posterior vaginal fornix by means of an Ayre spatula and smeared on to a clean glass slide, which is then immediately immersed in a fixing solution of alcohol and ether. After staining, these Papanicolau or cytology smears are examined under the microscope. Malignant cells have particular characteristics by which they can be recognized. The nuclei are large and irregular. Cervical smears are very accurate (98% correct) in the diagnosis of malignant disease of the cervix. Most gynæcologists would agree that this investigation should be performed on all women attending a gynæcological out-patient department, as well as yearly upon all married women regardless of their age. Carcinoma of the cervix is a preventable disease.

Treatment

The treatment for carcinoma of the cervix is:—
  (1) Radiotherapy.
  (2) Surgery.
  (3) Combination of both.

Radium has been used extensively for many years. It offers about as good a prospect of cure as surgery, and has a very low operative mortality, but may produce fibrosis in the pelvis which may involve rectum or bladder. The operation needed to eradicate carcinoma of cervix is an extensive one, with an operative mortality of about 5% in good hands, and 1-2% in the best hands. The decision between radiotherapy and surgery depends on the stage of the growth, the facilities available, and the views of the surgeon.

Radiotherapy

Though X-rays may be used post-operatively, or as a palliative treatment in advanced cases, radium is the most used form of radiotherapy. It is inserted in containers into the cervical canal and the vaginal fornices, and the dose required must be carefully calculated, as damage to the rectum is very easily done, and somewhat less easily to the bladder. There are several ways in which radium can be employed, but the Manchester technique is widely used, and is the one described here.

The patient is seen by the surgeon in consultation with the radiotherapist, and the dose agreed. Vaginal douches are given to clear infection, and the preparation of the patient for the radium insertion is the same as for an abdominal operation, and includes adequate emptying of the rectum. Under general anæsthesia and with the patient in the lithotomy position, a 20–35 mgm. radium container is inserted into the uterus, the dose depending on its size. Two or three plastic ovoids with 20 or 25 mgm. in each are put into the fornices; spacers are used to keep them apart, and a vaginal pack firmly inserted to retain the radium in position and keep the bladder and rectum from excessive radiation. The strings from the applicators are strapped to the thigh, and an X-ray picture taken to ensure a correct position. An indwelling catheter will be inserted into the bladder.

On the patient's return to the ward, the sister will sign a form for receipt of the radium, and will be given by the radium curator a lead box. An indicator, such as a red label, may be attached to the foot of the bed.

Radium is expensive, and can be dangerous in the wrong place, and with many methods of application elaborate precautions are necessary against loss. In this case the radium cannot be lost while the pack is in position, and such precautions are unnecessary. The patient must not be allowed out of bed, and each time the catheter spigot is released at three-hourly intervals, the fact that the pack and strings are in place should be checked. The patient is warned against touching the area.

Three or four days later the radium is removed in the ward, if necessary after the administration of morphine 16 mgm. The patient lies in the dorsal position with the knees flexed, and the sister will wear rubber gloves. She swabs and dries the vulva, and takes out the catheter. The pack is removed with a pair of forceps into a kidney dish lying on the bed. The strapping is taken off, and if

DISORDERS OF THE UTERUS

traction is made on the strings with a pair of pressure forceps, the radium will come out quite easily. With the strings held in the forceps, the radium is rinsed in a bowl of water, and put into the lead box. The radium curator signs for its receipt and takes it back to the radiotherapy department.

The second application will take place a week to ten days later, and during this time the patient will remain in the ward and undertake moderate activity. She may have a bath, but should kneel to avoid access of water to the vagina. The second stage of treatment is exactly like the first.

After the second stage is complete, the patient should spend a few days in the ward before going home. Though major reactions to radium are unusual, some nausea and anorexia may be felt, and it is also wise to have a full blood count done before discharge. Though radium application may seem minor compared with surgery for carcinoma of cervix, it is for the patient a time of anxiety and fatigue, and she needs both rest and encouragement.

If the surgeon feels that the procedure will increase the hope of cure, he may remove the lymph glands on the side wall of the pelvis—PELVIC LYMPHADENECTOMY. Alternatively, high voltage X-ray therapy may be used to treat them.

NURSING PATIENTS HAVING DEEP X-RAY THERAPY

Irradiation of the pelvis by deep X-rays is not uncommonly used as a prophylactic measure after hysterectomy and removal of the appendages for malignant disease, or a palliative course may be given for carcinoma of the ovary. The nursing problems are the same for all gynæcological patients.

Treatment is given both to the front and the back of the pelvis, and the care of the irradiated skin is of great importance. Soap and water must not be used, soap being especially irritating. The skin is best kept dry, and if reddening occurs starch powder may be dusted on. The nightdress should be of soft material, and a sorbo mattress or air ring will help to prevent soreness of the back.

If vaginal discharge is present, douches of warm water may be given at the discretion of the gynæcologist and careful and frequent toilet of the vulva practised. Pads should be supplied, frequently renewed, and they should be kept in place with a T-bandage of soft material, and not by a belt which will be tight enough to irritate the skin.

Nausea and vomiting are frequently troublesome, as in all cases when X-rays are being used on the abdomen. In spite of much research over many years, no reliable cure for radiation sickness is yet available, but there are several drugs worth trying. Chloretone gr. 10 is an old remedy, but one of the most reliable. Pyridoxin (vitamin B6) 50 mgm. a day, or ascorbic acid 100 mgm., twice a day may be effective, while the motion-sickness remedies like Dramamine and Avomine are often prescribed. The most important point from the nurse's point of view is to see that sickness does not unduly interfere with nutrition. Vomiting most commonly occurs after treatment; and if this is in the morning the patient may be unable to take lunch, which in hospital may be the main meal of the day. The nurse must make sure then that there is some high caloric addition to the other meals. Protein in adequate quantities must be given in the diet. If fat is badly tolerated, sugar must be given in such forms as honey or sweetened fruit juices. It is absolutely imperative to keep a fluid balance chart, and to see that it records not what the patient is offered, but what she is able to take.

Diarrhœa is common and very disturbing. Mist. Cretæ et Opii (chalk and opium mixture) 15 ml. ($\frac{1}{2}$ fl. oz.) four-hourly is often effective, or a starch and opium enema will sometimes ensure a restful night if it is given before the patient is settled to sleep. Four ounces of starch mucilage are given through a No. 8 catheter, and thirty or sixty minims of tincture of opium poured into the funnel when half the starch has run in. If the anus becomes sore, benzocaine ointment can be applied.

Cystitis may occur through irritation of the bladder by the X-rays. A high fluid intake must be maintained for this reason also, and an alkaline mixture will help to reduce the frequency of micturition.

No complaint should be disregarded, but imagination should be used to deal with symptoms as they arise, and thus encourage the patient to bear with fortitude the discomforts so often attendant on treatment.

DISORDERS OF THE UTERUS

Surgery

The operation most practised in this country to-day is Wertheim's hysterectomy. This entails the removal of all pelvic tissue except the bladder, ureters, rectum, great vessels and nerves, and enough peritoneum to cover the bare area.

The patient is admitted a week before operation for examination under anæsthesia, biopsy of the growth and cystoscopy, during which a specimen of urine will be taken for culture. Her consent and that of her husband to operation is obtained. The hæmoglobin percentage and blood group

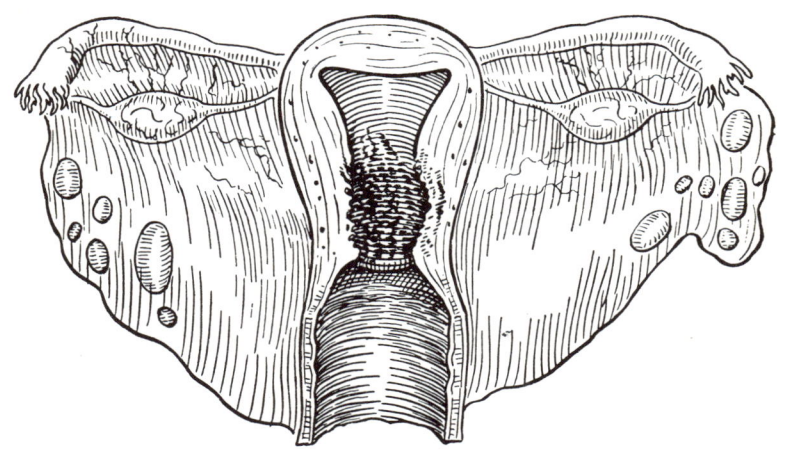

FIG. 51. Diagram to show the tissues removed by Wertheim's hysterectomy.

are ascertained and the chest X-rayed. The blood urea is estimated and an intravenous pyelogram performed to exclude involvement of the ureters in the growth.

A diet with plenty of protein is given and a high fluid intake encouraged. Vitamins B and C are of value pre- and post-operatively.

The pre-operative measures outlined in Chapter 3 are undertaken. An hour and a half before operation the patient passes urine, and the vagina is packed with penicillin gauze if the surgeon requests it. The following are needed:—

Sterile dish, with gauze roll two yards long and large gallipot.

Sterile sponge-holding forceps.
Penicillin 60 ml., 1,000 units per ml.
Sterile Sims' speculum or Landon's retractor.
Warm lotion and swabs.
Receiver for dirty dressings.
Blanket, mackintosh and towel.

The bed is screened, and the patient assured that after this she will be settled down to sleep until the operation. She is helped into the left lateral position, suitably covered, and the buttocks brought well to the edge of the bed. The insertion of such a pack needs skill, since it involves introducing a speculum, which may provoke bleeding, and filling the vagina with gauze, which can be uncomfortable and even painful. A good light is needed, and an assistant to hold the dish lest the pack become contaminated by touching the thigh before insertion. Sims' speculum can be used, but has a thin edge which may produce bleeding from the growth, and if it is available, Landon's retractor, which has a rounded margin, will be found preferable.

The operator washes her hands and swabs the vulva, the retractor is introduced, and the perineum drawn back, while the assistant pours the penicillin over the gauze roll. A generous amount of the pack should be gathered into the sponge-holding forceps, to avoid touching the growth with the instrument, and the gauze introduced along the retractor into the posterior fornix. The vault is packed first, and the whole vagina firmly but not tightly filled, and a sterile pad applied. The rest of the pre-operative routine with regard to gown, false teeth and pre-operative drug is completed, and the patient settled down to sleep.

In the anæsthetic room, the pack will be withdrawn and the bladder catheterized; a blood transfusion is begun, and the patient placed in the Trendelenburg position. Through a midline incision the uterus, tubes, ovaries, pelvic glands, cellular tissue lateral to the uterus, and the greater part of the vagina are removed. Adhesions may create difficulty, and the surgeon takes the greatest care to identify and preserve the ureters. A flavine and paraffin pack is inserted into the vagina, and a self-retaining catheter into the bladder, and connected to a sterile uribag.

In the ward her bed has been prepared and warmed, and blocks put ready at the foot. On a trolley is a treatment

DISORDERS OF THE UTERUS

board, thermometer, sphygmomanometer and a mouth tray.

On return to the ward, the patient's perineal pad is briefly inspected for bleeding, and the uribag inspected to ensure that the catheter is draining and the urine is not bloodstained. Her temperature, pulse and respiration are recorded, and the pulse should be charted every fifteen minutes. The blood pressure should be taken as required by the surgeon, and as soon as consciousness begins to return pethidine 100 mgm. or papaveretum 20 mgm. should be administered. The blood transfusion is regulated to the required rate. During the rest of the day of operation, attention is given to restoring the patient from the surgical shock so common after such a long operation. As her condition improves she is gradually sat up. On the next day she may begin to take fluids by mouth, but it is usually necessary to continue to give intravenous fluid. The usual care of the mouth and pressure points is given, and pain prevented by pethidine 100 mgm. six-hourly. The uribag is changed daily.

The intravenous infusion will usually be discontinued on the second day providing satisfactory bowel sounds are present and fluids given freely by mouth. Light solids can also be given, and most patients appreciate thin bread and butter or a biscuit rather than the semi-solid sweets or ice-cream so frequently offered. The pack is removed to-day, after morphine 16 mgm., and a sterile pad applied, as some watery bloodstained discharge can be expected. Subsequently the vulva must be swabbed three or four times daily to avoid sepsis in the vagina and urethra and to promote the patient's comfort. Abdominal distension will begin to be troublesome to-day, and will continue as peristalsis returns.

On the third day wound pain will be decreasing, and codeine tablets should suffice as an analgesic. Distension is now at its most troublesome, but peristalsis should be returning, and the surgeon may permit the passage of a flatus tube, or a glycerine suppository. If bowel sounds are not heard, or if there is vomiting, the possibility of paralytic ileus should be borne in mind, and the surgeon consulted immediately. If this unfortunate complication appears, fluids by mouth should be withheld and an intravenous infusion begun, continuous gastric aspiration through an indwelling Ryle's tube instituted, and morphine 10 mgm. will be prescribed four-hourly. If, however, all is well, the patient is lifted into an armchair, taking her uribag with her, while the bed is made.

Progress now should be continuous. The diet is increased to normal, and a paraffin emulsion can be given to aid bowel action. Activity in bed and out is slowly increased. A careful watch is still kept on the temperature and pulse, on the nature of the discharge, and on the urine. Pyrexia may mean vaginal infection, cystitis, thrombophlebitis at the intravenous site, or the more serious thrombosis of the leg veins. Slight fever should never be disregarded, but the cause actively sought and treated.

On the seventh day the clips may be removed from the abdominal wound, and the stitches on the next day. On the tenth day the catheter can be removed. The reason for the long continuation of bladder drainage is that the nerve supply to the bladder has inevitably been damaged, and in addition removal of pelvic tissue has left the bladder unsupported. The patient is unlikely to micturate naturally until healing has occurred. Following the removal of the catheter, the output and frequency must be recorded, and residual urine must not be allowed to accumulate. If the patient cannot pass urine, the catheter is replaced for forty-eight hours; if the residual urine is more than 400 ml. the catheter is replaced for forty-eight hours. Otherwise, the residual urine is estimated daily until it is less than 150 ml.

The possibility of secondary hæmorrhage still exists, but is less likely than in some other operations. After the fourteenth day there is less fear of any complication, and discharge to a convalescent home can be arranged, when the condition permits. Follow-up by the outpatient department will begin in a month's time.

The post-operative care of this patient has been described in some detail because it illustrates the attention to detail and the careful observation needed by the nurses in the gynæcological wards. Good nursing plays a vital part in preserving the patient's life in the initial post-operative phase, and may do a very great deal to alleviate the many discomforts attendant on it.

NURSING OF ADVANCED CARCINOMA OF CERVIX

A number of patients are still seen for the first time when the disease is far advanced, and there are others for whom treatment has been unable to stop the spread of the growth, and nursing care can do much to mitigate their discomfort. The patient is often emaciated, and should be nursed on a comfortable mattress, and have frequent attention paid to the pressure points. The appetite will be poor, and small attractively served meals should be offered. Spread into the bladder may cause pain and frequency of micturition, and the prescription of potassium citrate and hyoscyamus in addition to analgesics may be helpful. If the bladder wall is perforated, and a vesico-vaginal fistula results, incontinence of urine will occur, and the skin of the vulva will need protection by ointment, and cellulose pads, frequently changed, must be provided. Sometimes an indwelling catheter in the bladder, with continuous suction applied, is helpful. If it is not successful in keeping the patient dry, a second catheter may be put into the vagina and kept in place by a vaseline pack and both connected by a Y-tube to the sucker.

Recto-vaginal fistula may cause incontinence of fæces, and regular swabbing of the vulva and renewal of dressings is then necessary. The most constant symptom is the very offensive discharge, often heavily blood-stained. Irrigation of the vulva with a douche can and a soft rubber catheter, or pouring lotion from a jug over the vulva may be helpful and the groins and thighs should be washed with soap and water and powdered four-hourly when the pressure points are treated. Pads should be changed frequently, and if the smell is distressing deodorants can be used near the bed.

Pain should be relieved first with the simpler analgesics like codeine, later with pethidine and morphine. If the cancer involves the ureters, uræmia will supervene, and the vomiting which becomes such a distressing feature may be helped by the prescription of chlorpromazine, which may also have a helpful calming effect. Every symptom that arises should be considered as a nursing problem for which a solution should be sought.

MODERN GYNÆCOLOGY FOR NURSES
CARCINOMA OF THE BODY OF THE UTERUS

A typical patient with this disease might be sixty years old (though the disease is not confined to the older woman), rather overweight, giving a history of recent vaginal bleeding. This is the first symptom, and often leads the patient to seek medical advice early, since she recognizes bleeding after the menopause as abnormal. Offensive discharge and pain occur later.

The prospects of cure are better than in carcinoma of the cervix for the following reasons:—

(1) Cases are seen at a somewhat earlier stage.

(2) The growth is confined by the thick uterine wall, and does not infiltrate other structures for some time.

(3) The patients are usually of an age when the advance of malignant disease is at a slower rate.

Examination may disclose enlargement of the uterus, and not infrequently sugar will be found in the urine, since

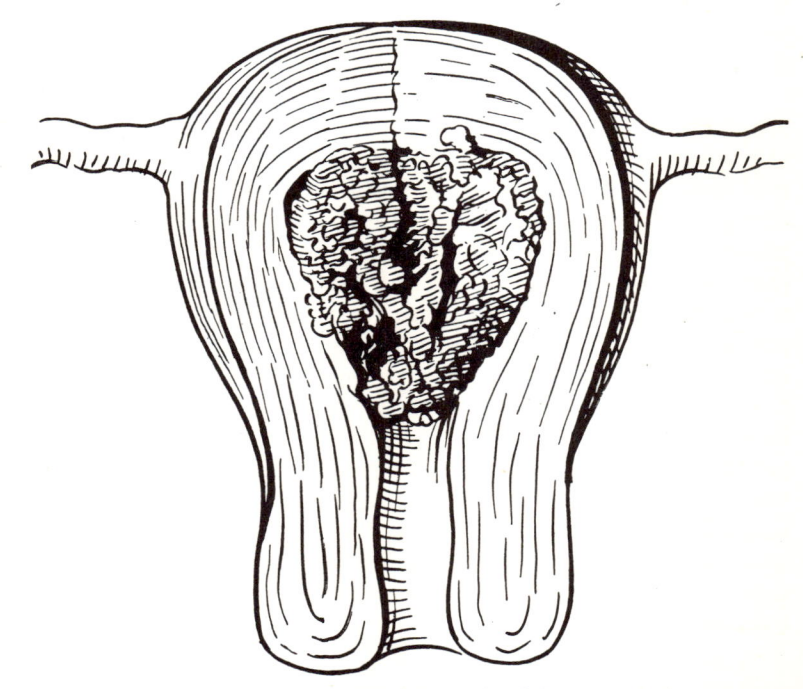

FIG. 52. Carcinoma of the body of the uterus.
Compare with Fig. 49.

DISORDERS OF THE UTERUS

a fair proportion of such women are diabetics. If no abnormality can be detected, a diagnostic dilatation and curettage of the uterus is undertaken. Under a general anæsthetic the cervix is dilated up to number 10 of Hegar's dilators, and the uterus carefully curetted, and the material sent for a pathological report. It is often possible to confirm the diagnosis at once by examination of the curettings, and to proceed immediately to the operation of choice, which is an extended abdominal total hysterectomy with removal of a good cuff of the upper vagina and bilateral salpingo-oöphorectomy. The nurse should ascertain if such a possibility exists, since pre-operative preparation would then include the treatment of the vagina described for a Wertheim's hysterectomy.

An indwelling catheter will not usually be needed after such an operation, and a vaginal pack will only be used if bleeding has been troublesome at operation. Abdominal distension may need treatment, and a watch should be kept for any vaginal discharge that might indicate infection, and foreshadow secondary hæmorrhage.

PROLAPSE

In order to understand prolapse of the uterus and vagina, it is essential first to consider the normal supports of these two organs. Nurses should understand that, while it is possible to have a prolapse of the vagina without a prolapse of the uterus, there is usually an associated descent of both these organs simultaneously but, for the purposes of description, the supports of each will be described separately.

The Uterus

This organ is supported primarily by the ligament called the cardinal, transverse or Mackenrodt's which runs from the cervix to the side wall of the pelvis. This ligament must not be considered as a simple structure since it is a very complex one with an anterior and posterior prolongation. The anterior runs from the cervix to the symphysis pubis under the bladder and supports this organ, while the posterior part of the transverse ligament runs backward under the utero-sacral folds from the cervix to the side of the sacrum and encircles the rectum. In this way, a triple-

Fig. 53 — Supports of the Cervix

Fig. 54 — Supports of the Vagina

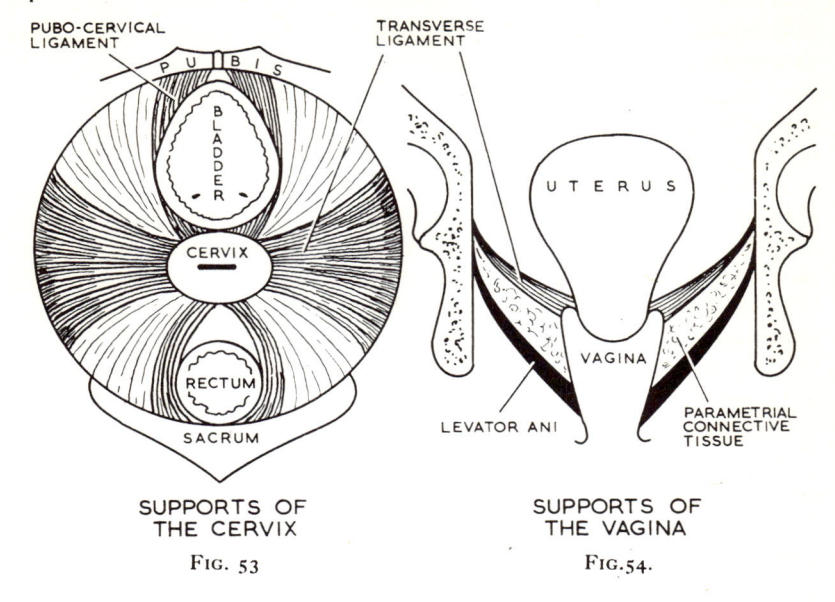

bodied ligament is formed and acts as a hammock which not only keeps the uterus from prolapsing but also helps to keep it anteverted and, at the same time, keeps the bladder in its correct position. The ligament which supports the bladder, that is the anterior part of the transverse cervical ligament, is frequently called the pubo-cervical ligament.

Cause of Prolapse. During the process of childbirth, the cervix dilates to allow the passage of the fœtal head and, as it dilates, the transverse ligament is carried upwards and to the sides of the pelvis. If the child is delivered either by precipitate labour or by forceps, before the cervix is fully dilated, the cervix will be pulled down by the fœtal head, like a skull-cap with a hole in the middle, and the supporting ligament will be irreparably damaged. When a woman has had a difficult confinement or a number of children, the transverse cervical ligament becomes increasingly weakened and the muscular structures in it become replaced with fibrous tissue which is never as strong as living muscle. Most cases of prolapse occur at or after the menopause because at this time all the ligaments and muscles in a woman's body tend to atrophy and increasing obesity causes a rise of intra-abdominal pressure and so there is a tendency for the uterus and vagina to be pushed

DISORDERS OF THE UTERUS

downwards. A chronic cough is also an important factor in causing or increasing a prolapse.

The Vagina

This structure is supported at its upper end by the transverse cervical ligament which has a broad attachment to the vaginal vault for at least a distance of half-way down it. At the junction of the middle two-thirds and the lower third of the vagina, the levatores ani are attached by a broad extension into the muscle of the vagina itself and the integrity of these muscles prevents the lower part of the vagina from prolapsing.

Causes of Prolapse. The extreme distension of the vagina by the child during its birth must always cause some tearing and disruption of the levatores ani which are pulled

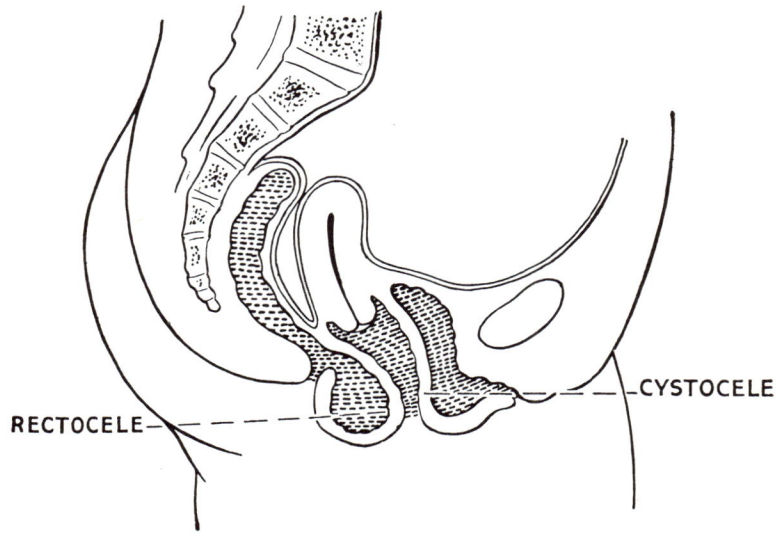

FIG. 55. Prolapse of the anterior and posterior vaginal walls, cystocele and rectocele.

to each side in the region of the perineal body and, in addition, the circular fibres of the vagina are themselves ruptured by the distension of the baby. As a result of this, a weak place is left where the rectum and vagina are in relation to each other, that is, in the middle third, and there is a tendency for the rectum to bulge through the posterior vaginal wall when the woman raises her intra-abdominal pressure, as in coughing; hence the importance of a chronic cough in the cause of prolapse. This bulge is called a RECTOCELE. Damage to the anterior vaginal wall, especially the ligament under the bladder (the pubo-cervical, already referred to), will allow the bladder to bulge downwards into the anterior wall of the vagina and this is called a CYSTOCELE. There is a third interesting type of vaginal prolapse in which the upper third of the posterior wall of the vagina, which is related to the anterior part of Douglas's pouch, becomes weakened, not always as a result of childbirth but sometimes in elderly spinsters of an asthenic type with poor muscular and ligamentary tone, and this is called a hernia of Douglas's pouch or an ENTEROCELE because it may contain some bowel. Sometimes an enterocele becomes herniated through the vulva and is usually mistaken for a rectocele with which it may be associated. The two conditions, however, are anatomically quite different.

Three degrees of uterine prolapse are described, which indicate approximately the amount of the descent. In the first, the cervix lies at a lower level than is normal; in the second, the cervix presents at the introitus; and in the third it lies outside the vaginal orifice. In PROCIDENTIA, the most extensive form of third degree prolapse, the whole uterus lies outside the body, having carried with it the vaginal walls which are turned inside out. If such a condition has been present for any length of time the vagina will be ulcerated from pressure, friction and irritation by the urine, and the patient will need careful preparation to cure the ulceration and the infection before the condition is treated, preferably by vaginal hysterectomy and repair of the prolapsed vagina and associated structures. The symptoms of prolapse depend on which structures have descended. Frequency of micturition, urinary infection and stress incontinence; difficulty in defæcation, vaginal discharge and an aching or dragging sensation in the perineum are common examples. In addition, backache and what the patient describes as intense weariness are almost universal complaints.

In the operative treatment of prolapse, surgeons endeavour, by making a careful dissection of the vagina from

DISORDERS OF THE UTERUS

the bladder in front and from the rectum behind, to reconstitute the muscles and the ligaments which support these structures and to replace them in the position in which they were before the patient became pregnant. A description of these complicated operations is not within the scope of this book but one important step should be emphasized, namely, the dissection of the levators in their laterally displaced position in the pelvis and the suture of the levatores together in the midline to reform the muscular pelvic floor which supports the vagina and, for that matter, all the contents of the female pelvis. Incompetence of the leva-

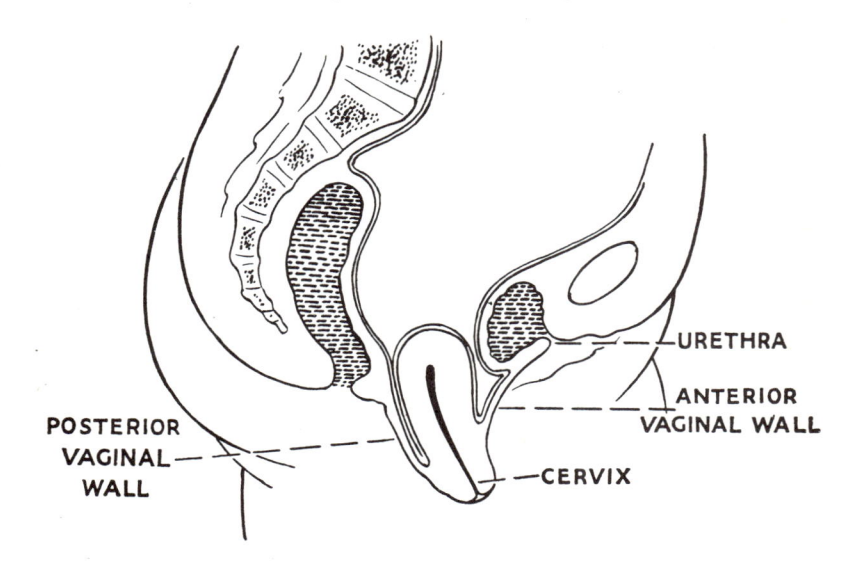

FIG. 56. Procidentia, or complete prolapse of the uterus, which lies outside the body.

tores is like opening two swing doors by pushing them in front of you and this opening allows the passage through the doors of whatever may be pressing from behind—in this case the uterus, bladder and rectum. One further problem of prolapse which is important is that of STRESS INCONTINENCE. In this condition, the control of urine when the intra-abdominal pressure is raised is impaired and, if the patient coughs, sneezes, laughs or even exerts herself like running for a bus, she is liable to eject a small quantity of urine down her urethra and this is called stress incontinence. It is caused by damage to the specialized smooth muscle at the neck of the bladder or alteration of the angle between the urethra and the bladder neck.

It is an extremely common symptom in women who have borne children and is probably present in 50% of all cases of prolapse of the anterior vaginal wall. It is often associated with a bulge of the urethra into the lower half of the vagina when the woman strains and this is called a URETHROCELE. The treatment of this condition is complicated and the results not always satisfactory, but the aim of the surgeon is to repair the smooth muscle and the angle at the junction of the bladder and the urethra and to repair the fascia of the pubo-cervical ligament underneath the weak spot. This operation is called the anterior colporrhaphy and involves some repair of the supports of the bladder as well. The repair of the posterior vaginal wall is called a posterior colporrhaphy. These two operations are usually done together and may be associated with amputation of the cervix if it is diseased, elongated or hypertrophied. When this operation is performed, it is always associated with some repair to the transverse ligament which is shortened and transplanted in front of the lower part of the uterus just above the amputated cervix. This operation is called a Manchester or Fothergill's operation and is the most commonly employed operation for uterine prolapse which a nurse will see. If the uterus itself is diseased or if the woman is complaining of severe symptoms such as menorrhagia, or if the uterus contains small fibroids, an anterior and posterior colporrhaphy is combined with a vaginal hysterectomy and this operation is called a vaginal hysterectomy and repair or the Mayo-Ward operation.

POST-OPERATIVE NURSING

Following an operation for prolapse, the nursing management will be on the following lines. The patient's general condition should be good, but sometimes there has been some blood loss, especially if vaginal hysterectomy has been performed, in which case a blood transfusion will be given. An indwelling catheter is usually in place, and if there has been any difficulty in hæmostasis there will be a pack in the vagina. The nurse looks at the vulval pad to see if there is any loss, removes the spigot from the catheter and connects it to a uribag. As the patient begins to recover consciousness, she is given an analgesic, such as morphine 10 mg. or pethidine 100 mg., and is raised into a semi-recumbent position, with a foam ring under the buttocks.

If the anterior vaginal wall has not been repaired, the surgeon may omit the indwelling catheter, in the hope that the patient may micturate normally. If she cannot do so readily without straining, a Foley catheter should be passed.

On the day after operation, fluids and light solids can be given, and the patient is encouraged to drink freely. Pethidine will usually be required today and perhaps the next for pain. Although cystocele causes more troubles before operation than rectocele, after operation it is posterior wall repair that causes most discomfort. After 48 hours a codeine mixture, or soluble aspirin or paracetamol will suffice.

Toilet of the perineum is begun on the first day. The pad is removed, and swabs moistened in cetrimide or savlon and held in forceps are used to clean the vulva and the perineal stitches. The catheter is also cleaned of any dried secretion. This should be done two or three times a day until the patient is able to take a bath, usually a few days after operation. The pack is removed after 48 hours; if it were by mischance forgotten infection of the vaginal stitchline and secondary bleeding might follow.

Breathing exercises should be begun soon after operation. Pneumonia is not common after this operation, unless the patient has a chronic cough, but deep breathing will increase diaphragmatic movement, which by drawing on the inferior vena cava will encourage venous return from the calves, and so lessen the risk of venous thrombosis in the legs. The patient may be helped out of bed for a short time on the first day, and this will also help the circulation.

It is common to leave the catheter in the bladder for a week, putting a spigot in the catheter after 48 hours and releasing it at intervals. Nitrofurantoin 100 mgm. t.d.s. is ordered to prevent urinary infections. A specimen of urine is put up daily, and the output is measured. When the catheter is removed, a close watch must be kept on the output, and the frequency. It is difficult to empty the bladder at first (i.e. there is residual urine), but this usually rights itself. If the patient can pass no urine, or if she passes very small quantities at short intervals (suggesting retention with overflow), a catheter is put into the bladder for a further 48 hours.

The bowels are kept confined for a few days, especially if posterior colporrhaphy has been performed, in order to allow the suture lines to heal. A non-bulky diet is taken until the bowels are open. An aperient such as Milpar can be given on the third or fourth evening, and if a bowel action is not secured on the following morning, a glycerine suppository can be given.

The perineal stitches should be inspected daily. They are usually of catgut, and should dissolve away, but some surgeons like any remaining sutures removed on the 6th day. Œdema of the perineum sometimes occurs, and the tension on the suture line causes great discomfort, and removal of a stitch may help.

A rise of temperature indicates inflammation or infection. The nurse should examine the urine; the calf muscles for signs of tenderness that may mean thrombosis; consider the possibility of chest infection, and notice the nature of any vaginal discharge.

An offensive discharge, or obvious infection of those sutures that are visible, must be dealt with promptly. Infection may spread to the connective tissue in the pelvis, causing *parametritis*, and if not checked this may go on to cause pelvic abscess. A swab should be taken, and the organism and its antibiotic sensitivities ascertained, so that the appropriate drug can be given without delay. Twice daily baths are helpful. Local treatment is not usually advocated, but some surgeons may order vaginal irrigations, given through a soft catheter, at very low pressure, to avoid spreading infection upwards.

If infection is not dealt with, blood vessels may be opened up by the inflammatory process, and secondary hæmorrhage may occur in the second week. This used to be one of the most feared complications of vaginal surgery, but is now comparatively rarely seen. If of any magnitude it is treated by packing the vagina with dry gauze under anæsthetic in the theatre. A practical point is that menstruation may occur after colporrhaphy, so not all bleeding is pathological. The patient is usually ready for discharge

DISORDERS OF THE UTERUS

within a fortnight, depending on her general and local condition, and where she is going. Convalescence is desirable, as women quickly get involved in housework. An explanation of the operation should be given to the husband as well as the wife. If she is below the age of the menopause and the uterus is still intact, conception is possible. Intercourse is forbidden for six weeks, and the patient must avoid physical strain, such as is involved in lifting, or moving heavy articles, for about the same time. She should be given an appointment to see the surgeon in a month's time for assessment of the success of the operation.

Retroversion

Definition. A backward displacement of the uterus into Douglas's pouch from its normal anteverted position. This may be associated with retroflexion.

Types, Congenital and Acquired

Congenital Retroversion. Many women, especially those who suffer from genital hypoplasia, have a congenitally retroverted uterus. It causes no symptoms and requires no treatment and they would be better if they never knew about it. It is discovered only at routine pelvic examination.

Acquired Retroversion. This is almost always the result of subinvolution following abortion or childbirth although a few cases may be the result of pelvic inflammatory disease, usually in the tubes or ovaries, in which adhesions and fibrosis form around the inflammatory process and bind the uterus down in the retroverted position. This is the so-called fixed retroversion and is usually an indication for abdominal operation, not only to correct the retroversion, but also to deal with the associated pelvic inflammatory disease. Some cases of endometriosis of the ovary are also associated with retroversion.

The symptoms of retroversion are not all those of the displaced body of the uterus : (1) Menorrhagia. Owing to the chronic congestion of the uterus and ovaries, excessive menstrual bleeding is an occasional sign. (2) Congestive dysmenorrhoea: for the same reason. (3) Backache: felt in the middle of the sacrum, probably due to uterine con-

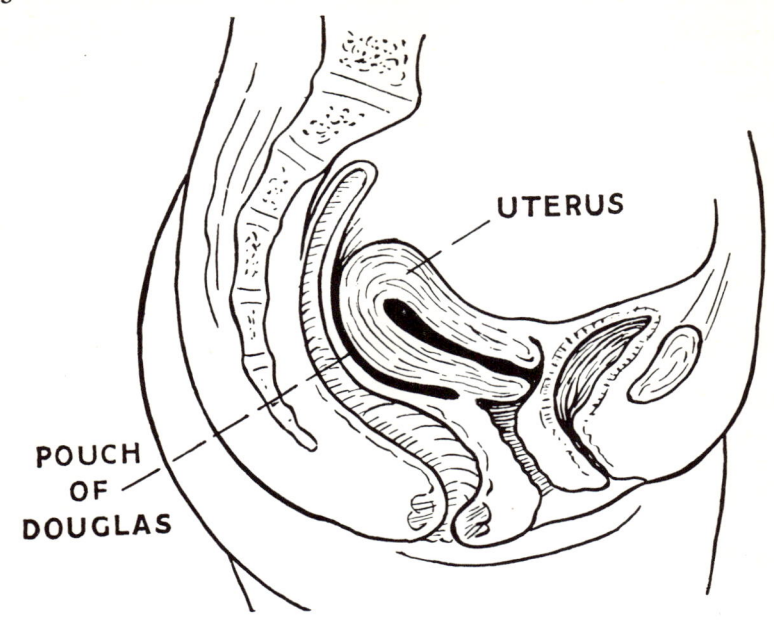

FIG. 57. Retroversion of the uterus. The fundus lies in the pouch of Douglas.

gestion. (4) Discharge. (5) Infertility. Some patients with retroversion suffer from impaired fertility because of the simple fact that the tubes are blocked: the retroversion does not of itself cause infertility. (6) Dyspareunia. This is pain on intercourse. The ovaries, when prolapsed with the uterus into the pouch of Douglas, may be exquisitely tender on bimanual examination and cause pain during intercourse. (7) The possibility that the pregnant uterus may become incarcerated in the pelvis at the fourteenth week and be unable to get out of it; this causes distortion and elongation of the urethra and leads to retention of urine. This is a rare but serious complication of the retroverted organ.

The presence of one or several of these symptoms is usually considered an indication for operation.

Operations. Sometimes in young women some form of suspension operation is performed. These operations are performed by the abdominal route and may be combined with other gynæcological procedures. In women nearer the menopause who desire no further children and where

DISORDERS OF THE UTERUS

the retroversion is associated with menorrhagia, backache, dyspareunia, etc., the best operation is a total hysterectomy. Sometimes in young women or those who are in the middle of their child-bearing period and in whom further conceptions are likely or desired, the uterus is manipulated, with or without an anæsthetic, into the anteverted position and held there temporarily by a Hodge pessary. If this relieves her symptoms, and they then recur after the Hodge pessary is removed, the surgeon is reasonably confident that surgical correction of the retroversion will also cure the symptoms. Finally, as stated above, a fixed retroversion associated with chronic pelvic inflammatory disease is almost always an indication for laparotomy.

SUPPORTIVE PESSARIES

The modern tendency is against the use of pessaries to support a prolapse, and very few women are too old or too frail to withstand an operation with the anæsthetic techniques of to-day. Not all the symptoms associated with

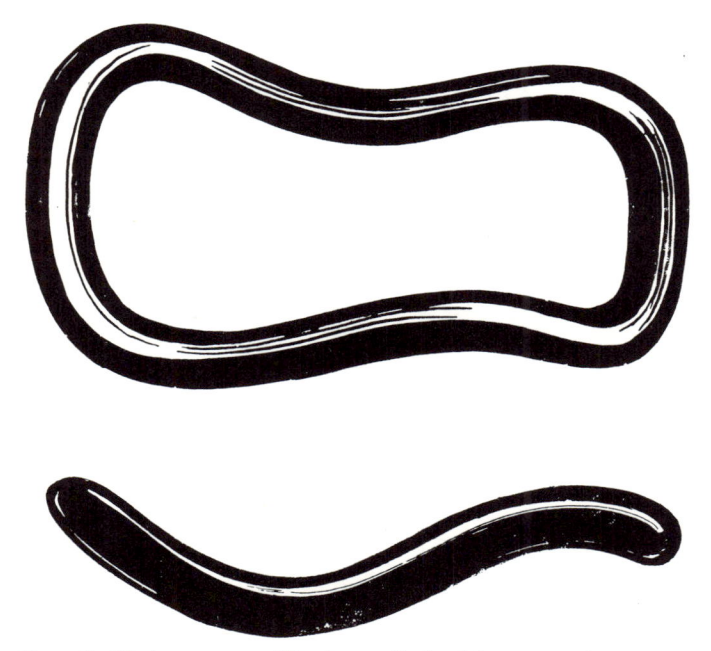

Fig. 58. Hodge pessary. The longer limb of the pessary lies behind the uterus to support it in the anteverted position.

prolapse can be cured by their use. Most women find the idea of such an appliance distasteful, to say the least, and the routine associated with its use is arduous.

The indications for prescribing a pessary are as follows:—

(1) Retroversion in the circumstances mentioned above; a Hodge pessary may be inserted by a doctor after correction of the retroversion. It is purely a temporary and diagnostic procedure.

(2) A general disease that will not permit any elective operation, e.g. active tuberculosis or heart failure.

(3) Refusal to have an operation.

(4) Prolapse occurring in a young woman after her first baby, if she is likely and anxious to conceive again. In this case a ring pessary may be used as a temporary stopgap until the desired family has been achieved. A properly performed prolapse operation is not, however, necessarily damaged by further childbirth, if a generous episiotomy is performed in labour (see p. 247).

(5) There may be a waiting period before admission to hospital for a prolapse operation, and during this time the woman may be kept symptom-free by a suitable pessary. Ring pessaries used to be made of rubber with a watch-

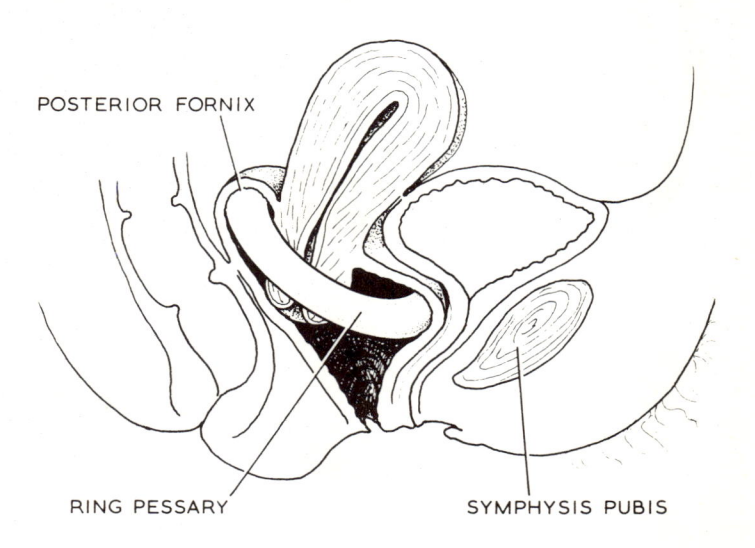

FIG. 59. Ring Pessary *in situ*.

DISORDERS OF THE UTERUS

spring core. A size must be selected that is large enough to control the prolapse, but not big enough to cause pain. A variety of plastic pessaries is now available, and these have the advantage of being less irritant to the vagina, and therefore less likely to cause a foreign-body vaginitis. They are easier to clean, and more compressible, and therefore more easily inserted and removed. The patient lies in the left lateral position, suitably covered. The nurse lubricates the ring with a little dettol cream or similar preparation, and may need to swab the vulva with lotion before insertion. Wearing gloves, with the left hand she parts the labia, and with the right compresses the ring firmly, and introduces it over the perineum into the vagina and releases it. With the first two fingers of the right hand, she pushes one edge of the ring into the anterior fornix, and then the opposite edge into the posterior fornix. The cervix should project through the ring, which should fit well and should support the prolapse efficiently.

The most important instruction to the patient is that she must have the plastic pessary changed every three months. Unhygienic or absent-minded patients are apt to keep a pessary in the vagina for long periods, even years. Such a retained foreign body can cause one of the foulest discharges met with in gynæcological practice.

The patient is also told that she must give herself a vaginal douche if there is a discharge, but this is not common with a plastic pessary. If the patient is an old lady who cannot undertake this for herself, the district nurse will help. All rings set up a vaginitis of greater or less degree, and all can, if neglected, cause a pressure ulceration.

INVERSION OF THE UTERUS

Inversion means the turning inside out of the uterus, and is the least frequently seen of all the uterine displacements. Acute inversion is only seen after delivery, and is almost invariably due to attempts to expel the placenta before it has become detached from the uterine wall, either by pressure on the fundus or by traction on the cord. The patient passes into a state of severe shock, the uterus can no longer be felt from the abdomen, and its interior presents at the vaginal orifice. It can usually be successfully re-

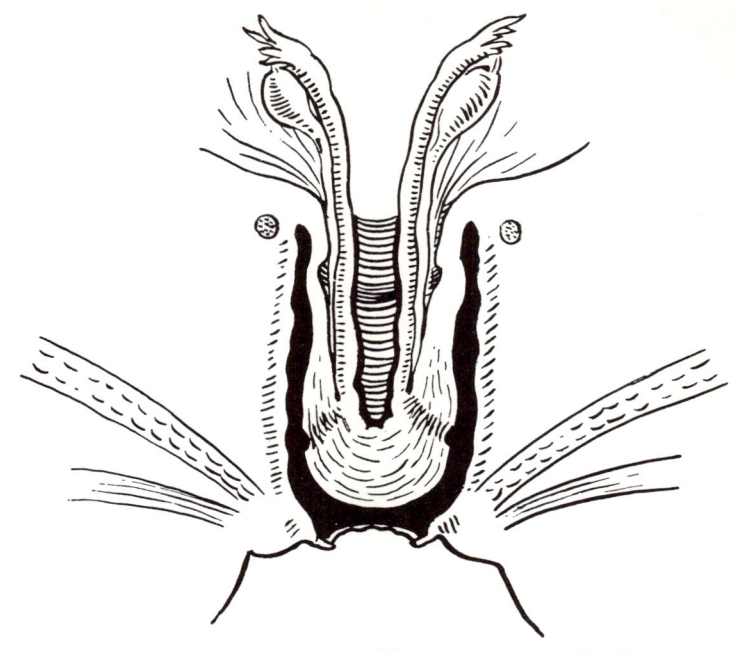

FIG. 60. Inversion of the uterus. The uterus is turned inside out, so that the interior of the fundus is the lowest presenting part.

placed immediately by simple manual replacement, or by filling the vagina with fluid under pressure, and with an anæsthetic. Blood transfusion and all anti-shock measures are indicated, and a course of chemotherapy should be begun to avert infection.

Chronic inversion of the uterus is sometimes caused by a fibroid polypus in the fundus being extruded by the uterus which turns itself inside out in the process. Such cases would to-day be treated by vaginal hysterectomy, unless there were some strong contra-indication to the loss of the uterus.

CHAPTER 8

DISEASES OF THE VAGINA AND VULVA

The vagina is the passage between the uterus and external genitalia. Its anterior wall, 9 cm. ($3\frac{1}{2}$ in.) in length, is related to the bladder in its upper part and the urethra in

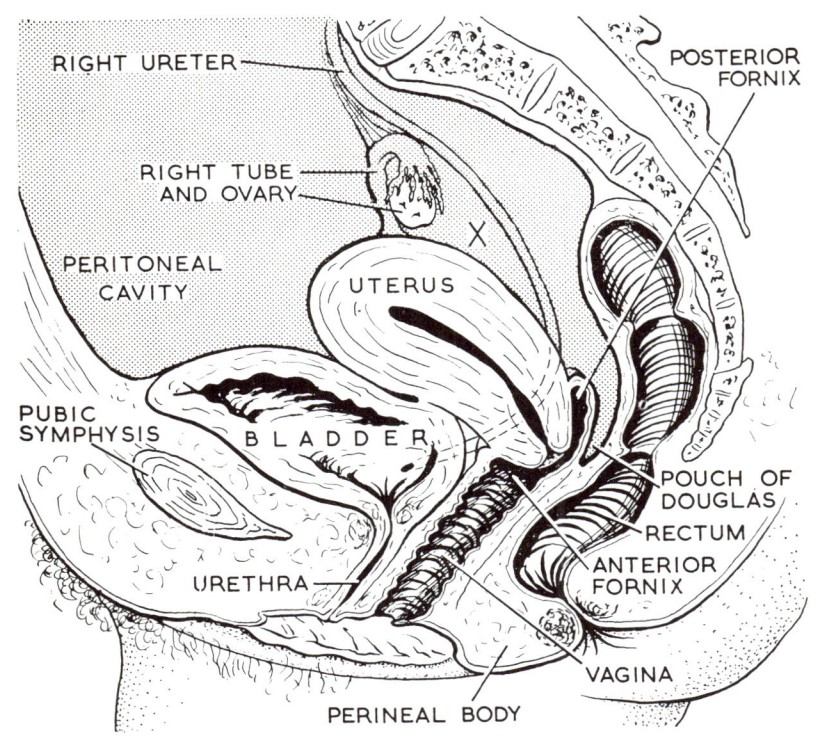

Fig. 61. The vagina and its relations.

the lower, while the posterior wall, which is 11 cm. ($4\frac{1}{2}$ in.) long, is in relation with the pouch of Douglas in its upper part, the rectum in the middle, and the perineal body in its lower third. It slants backwards from the orifice towards the **promontory** of the sacrum, an important point to remember when introducing a speculum. The vault of the vagina, into which the cervix projects, is divided into the anterior, posterior and two lateral fornices. Its supports have already been discussed in the section on prolapse.

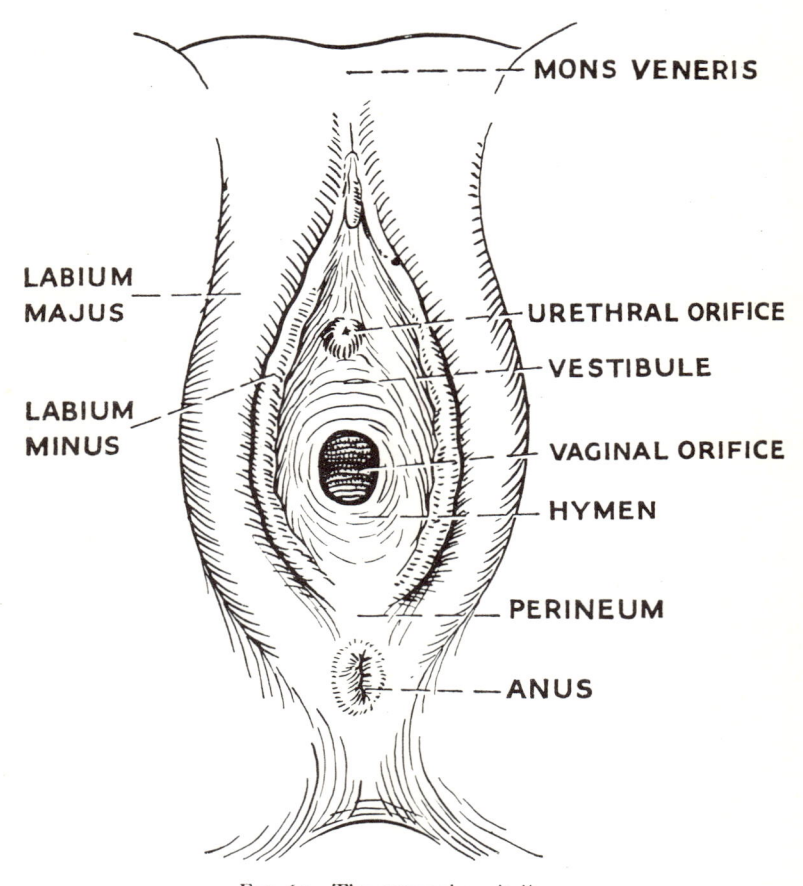

FIG. 62. The external genitalia.

Its lining is of stratified epithelium, and during the reproductive period of life, glycogen is present in the vaginal cells owing to the action of œstrogen. The vagina is not sterile, but the range of organisms in health is small, owing to the presence of Döderlein's bacillus, which ferments the glycogen and produces lactic acid. The high acidity of the vagina is its main protection against infection. Before

DISEASES OF THE VAGINA AND VULVA

puberty and after the menopause the concentration of acid is much less, or may be absent, so that young girls and elderly women are particularly susceptible to infection of the vagina.

The vulva is composed of the following structures:—

(1) The mons veneris, a cushion of fat lying over the symphisis pubis.

(2) The labia majora, two folds of skin and fat covered with hair.

(3) The labia minora, which are two thinner folds which divide anteriorly and enclose the clitoris.

(4) The clitoris, the female homologue of the penis, a small sensitive erectile organ.

(5) The vaginal orifice lies between the labia minora, partially closed in young girls by a fold of membrane, the hymen. The triangular space extending from the clitoris to the vaginal orifice is called the vestibule, and the opening of the urethra lies within it.

(6) Bartholin's glands are two mucous glands lying beneath the labia majora, and opening by a narrow duct onto the inner side of the labia minora, to which they provide a lubricant.

Infections of the Vagina

Vulvo-Vaginitis of little girls is often gonococcal in origin but may be streptococcal, and is described in the chapter on venereal disease. It is fortunately a condition which shows a marked decline.

Trichomonas vaginitis is a common condition caused by a protozoon, trichomonas vaginalis. The patient complains of an offensive and profuse discharge, which not only embarrasses her by its odour, but produces a secondary inflammation of the vulva. The appearance of the frothy yellowish discharge and its musty smell are characteristic, but in order to establish the diagnosis it is necessary to demonstrate the organism, and examination of a drop of fluid under the microscope discloses it moving by means of its flagella. It may reach the vagina from the rectum, or may be transmitted during intercourse.

The most efficient way of treating trichomonas infections is by giving the patient Flagyl (metronidazole) by mouth,

200 mgm. t.d.s. for seven days. Men develop a trichomonas urethritis, which is self-curing in three weeks. In order to avoid reinfection it is necessary to treat the husband as well as the patient.

Trichomonasidal pessaries may be used. It is important to ensure that the patient understands the correct method of insertion, since the pessary must be placed in the posterior fornix, and is quite inadequate if merely put into the lower part of the vagina. A pessary must be inserted last thing at night for six weeks, and treatment must be continued during menstruation for the three subsequent periods.

Thrush can occur in the vagina due to infection by a mould, candida albicans. It is most common during preg-

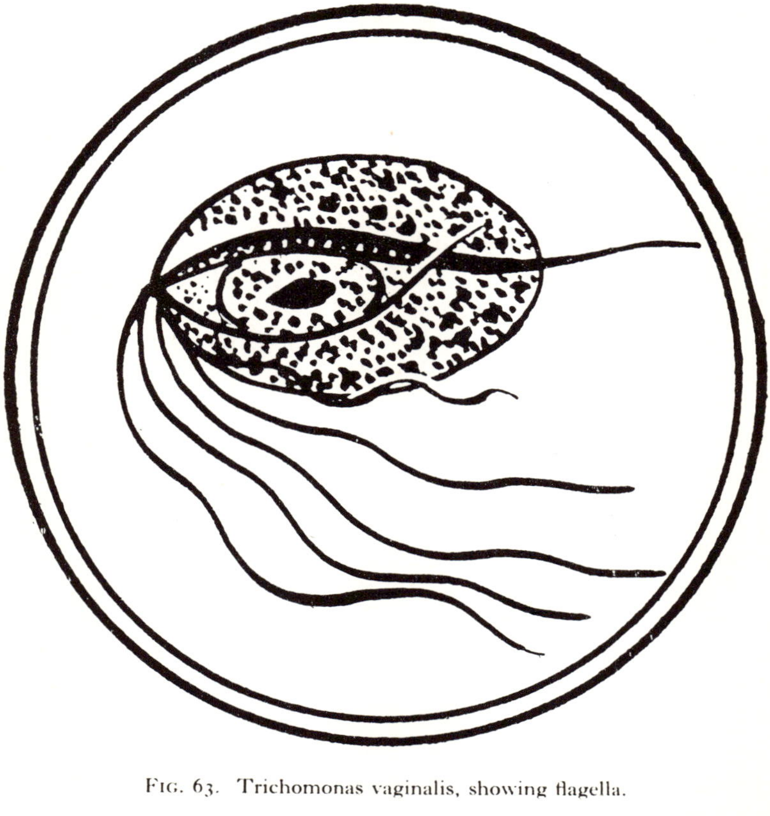

FIG. 63. Trichomonas vaginalis, showing flagella.

DISEASES OF THE VAGINA AND VULVA

nancy, may occur after a course of antibiotics, and is also common in diabetics, so that urine testing must never be omitted in such a case. Examination with a speculum shows dense, white, cheesy patches on the vaginal walls, sometimes extending to the vulva, and it causes a thick, creamy discharge and irritation.

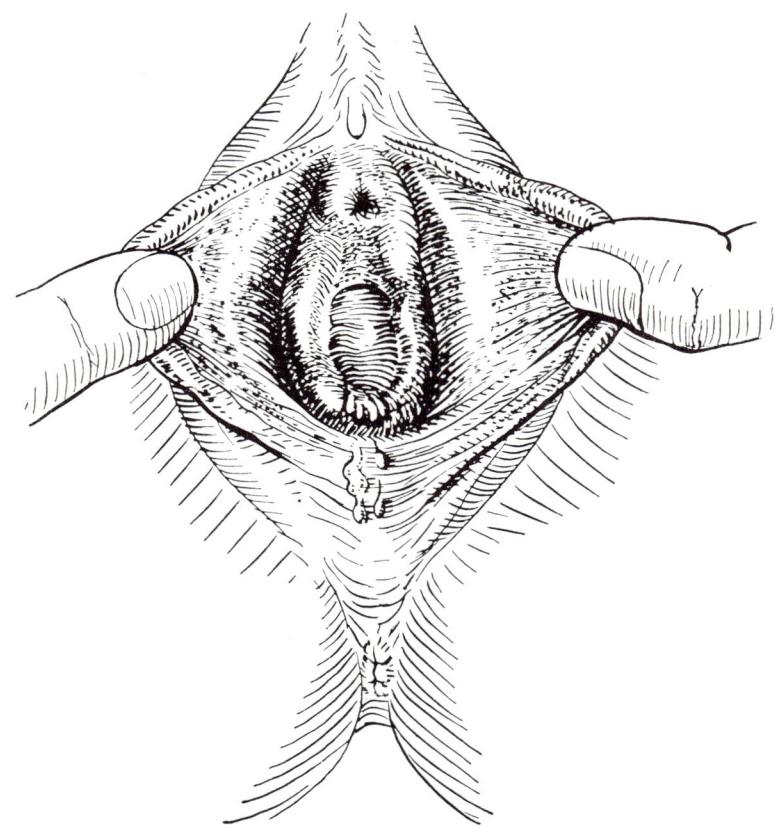

FIG. 64. Thrush of the vulva. White patches are seen on the inner surface of the labia minora and in the vestibule.

Nystatin and sporostacin are antibiotics that are active against thrush, and one pessary nightly for a fortnight will usually effect a cure, though a second course may be necessary. Resistant strains do not occur. An older treatment can be used, which consists of painting the vagina on alternate days with an aqueous solution of gentian violet 1%.

Gauze-covered swabs held in sponge-holding forceps should be used with a Cusco's or Sims' speculum and a good light. The patient lies in the left lateral position, the speculum is inserted, and if semi-solid material is seen in the vault of the vagina, it is removed with dry swabs. The whole of the cervix and vagina are then carefully and completely painted with the gentian violet. A pad should be supplied, and the patient is warned that the underclothing may be stained by the dye unless care is taken. Treatment is usually needed for about three weeks, and should be continued for a week after menstruation. If there is sugar in the urine this must be controlled if a cure is to be effected.

Senile or post menopausal vaginitis occurs in those women whose vaginal secretion loses its protective acid reaction after the menopause. The walls of the vagina are reddened, and show minute ulcers, and the discharge may become bloodstained. A vaginal swab should be taken for culture. It can always be cured by giving œstrogen, which restores the normal acidity and flora of the vagina. The œstrogen may be given locally as œstrogen cream inserted at night for three weeks, or by mouth (as stilbœstrol mgm. 0·05 daily for three weeks, or Premarin mgm. 0·625 once daily for two weeks) but it is important to remember that a prolonged course of oral œstrogen may cause uterine bleeding when it is stopped. Sometimes an antibiotic may be combined with the œstrogen pessary. Such œstrogen-withdrawal bleeding may cause difficulty in diagnosis, and the patient has to have a curettage to prove that such bleeding is not due to cancer of the uterus.

New growths of the vagina are uncommon, whether innocent or malignant. Secondary deposits from a **chorion epithelioma** (p. 236) may occur, and carcinoma of the cervix frequently extends into it, or carcinoma of the body or of the ovary may metastasize to the vagina, but primary growths are rare.

DISEASES OF THE VULVA

The vulva may be attacked by any of the conditions that affect the skin in general, such as boils or herpes. Boils in this area are painful and apt to occur in series. A single one should be treated in the same way as boils elsewhere, with special emphasis on frequent use of soap and water for the

DISEASES OF THE VAGINA AND VULVA

surrounding skin. If the boils are multiple, or appear in series, the labia may be shaved for greater ease in treating and cleaning the skin, and a course of an appropriate antibiotic can be given, together with a local antiseptic cream such as hibitane. Ultra-violet light, and the preparation of an autogenous vaccine are also useful measures in chronic cases.

Intertrigo is a maceration of the skin found where folds are in constant contact and moisture is present. It is only present in fat women, and is cured by strict attention to local cleanliness and dryness, and loss of weight.

Secondary vulvitis is often seen when a vaginal discharge is present which irritates the vulva, and such a secondary inflammation will not be cured till the cause is removed. Local treatment depends on the nature of the lesion, and whether the surface is weeping or infected. Antiseptic powders, lotions like lead lotion and aniline dyes like Bonney's blue are all useful. Ointments may be prescribed, but in general tend to make the skin sodden. If micturition is painful, the urine may be kept alkaline by potassium citrate. Sedatives are valuable, since itching is a common symptom, and will induce scratching, which still further injures the skin.

Sugar in the urine, as in diabetes mellitus, is especially liable to cause vulvitis, and very severe irritations are sometimes seen in women not previously known to be diabetic. Not only is the sugary urine irritating in itself, but organisms especially monilia grow readily on the moist skin sodden with glucose.

Leukoplakia is a chronic inflammatory condition of the skin, and is of importance because it is a pre-cancerous condition. It is sometimes seen on the tongue, but the most common site is the vulva, where it affects the labia majora and minora and sometimes the perineum, but not the vaginal orifice or urethra. Irritation is the first symptom, and arises about the time of the menopause. The skin is dry, red, tender and swollen, and later white patches appear, which in a severe case may cover the whole vulva. Cracks, which become very painful, may appear in the skin and malignant degeneration may follow.

Once the diagnosis has been made with certainty, the treatment for this undoubtedly pre-malignant condition is

144 MODERN GYNÆCOLOGY FOR NURSES

simple vulvectomy. The operation is not a severe one, and post-operative nursing presents no problems except the toilet of the wound with regard to micturition and defæcation. X-rays and œstrogenic drugs have been used as palliative measures, but are of no value and may be actually harmful.

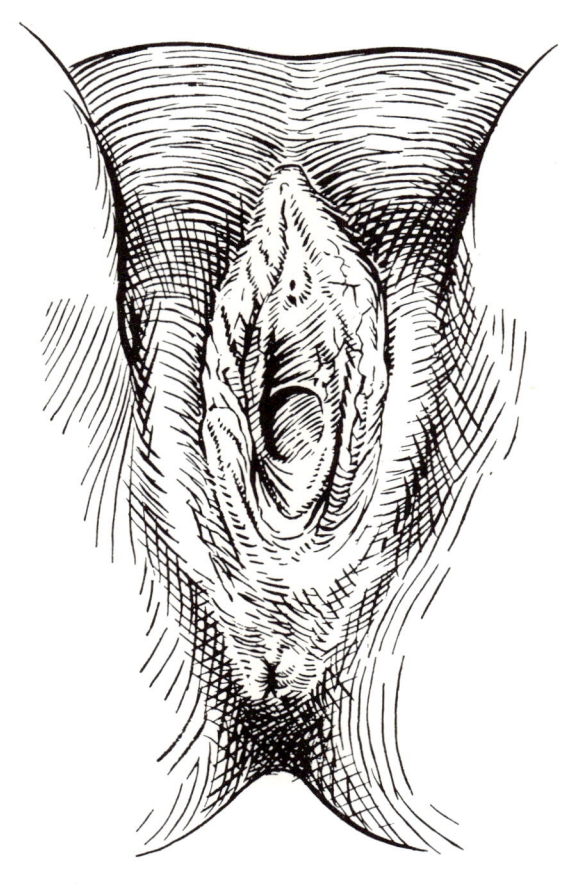

Fig. 65. Leukoplakia. The labia are whitened, and pre-malignant fissures are beginning to appear.

If malignant change has already taken place, the operation should be the radical one described for carcinoma of the vulva.

DISEASES OF THE VAGINA AND VULVA

Kraurosis is an atrophic condition, affecting especially the vestibule, and occurs at the time of the menopause. It is not malignant. There are small cherry-red patches, and the vulval epithelium is thinned out and transparent. Subepithelial infection and fibrosis develops later, with scarring and narrowing of the vaginal orifice, and dyspareunia is a common symptom. Since it is due to a fall in œstrogen secretion, it can be cured by oral stilbœstrol 0·1 mgm. daily, or ethinyl œstradiol 0·005 mgm. daily for three weeks. An œstrogen as an ointment for local application is useful, and analgesics are prescribed for the pain.

Urethral caruncle is a small granuloma (i.e. mass of granulation tissue) arising from the external urethral orifice. It is dark red in colour, bleeds very easily, and is extremely tender. It is treated by diathermy excision. An

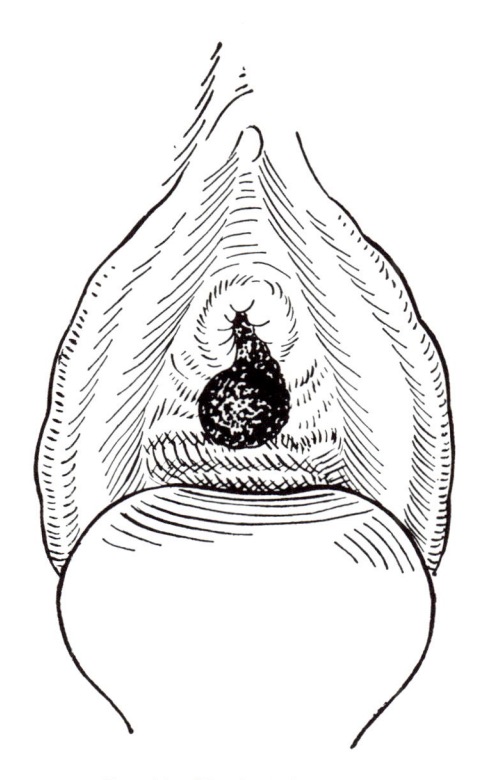

Fig. 66. Urethral Caruncle.

indwelling catheter is sometimes necessary after operation. If the patient has an associated kraurosis it is treated at the same time in the way described above.

Pruritus Vulvæ. Pruritus, or itching of the vulva, is a very common symptom in gynæcology. In a great many cases an obvious cause is present; it is frequently present in cases of vulvitis associated with a vaginal discharge and is a presenting symptom in leukoplakia. In other cases, the cause may be more difficult to establish. Conditions such as thread worms or hæmorrhoids may be the cause of irritation spreading forward from the anal region. In a few patients no cause can be found, and these are spoken of as idiopathic. The irritation is then thought to be the manifestation of a neurosis. Such a label is not used until the most searching clinical investigation fails to reveal a reason for the itching.

The pruritus is often worse just before menstruation, and may be troublesome during pregnancy, or most frequently of all at the menopause. It is usually worst at night when the patient is warm and has nothing to distract her from the irritation. She may be able to refrain from scratching by day, but not at night.

The cause of the irritation must be sought and treated, and examination of the urine must never be omitted. If no cause is found, the next most important point is to prevent the scratching, which produces hyperæmia of the vulva, and so increases the irritation and leads to more scratching. Adequate sedation at night is vital, and if the patient scratches in her sleep she should wear cotton gloves at night. Strict local cleanliness is necessary, with careful drying of the skin after washing. If the skin is excoriated, weeping or infected, the advice of the skin specialist should be asked, since the condition may be eczema, which soap would exacerbate. Hydrocortisone acetate ointment or one of its many variants is very successful in reducing inflammation or allaying irritation. Simple cooling lotions may be ordered. As a last resort, simple vulvectomy may have to be performed, and will cure the irritation, though if this is a manifestation of a personality disorder, symptoms elsewhere may be expected. Severe pruritus causes the most intense mental as well as physical distress, and much patience and tack will be needed in treatment.

DISEASES OF THE VAGINA AND VULVA 147

Bartholin's cyst is due to blocking of the duct that drains the gland, and at first the only sympton is a swelling.

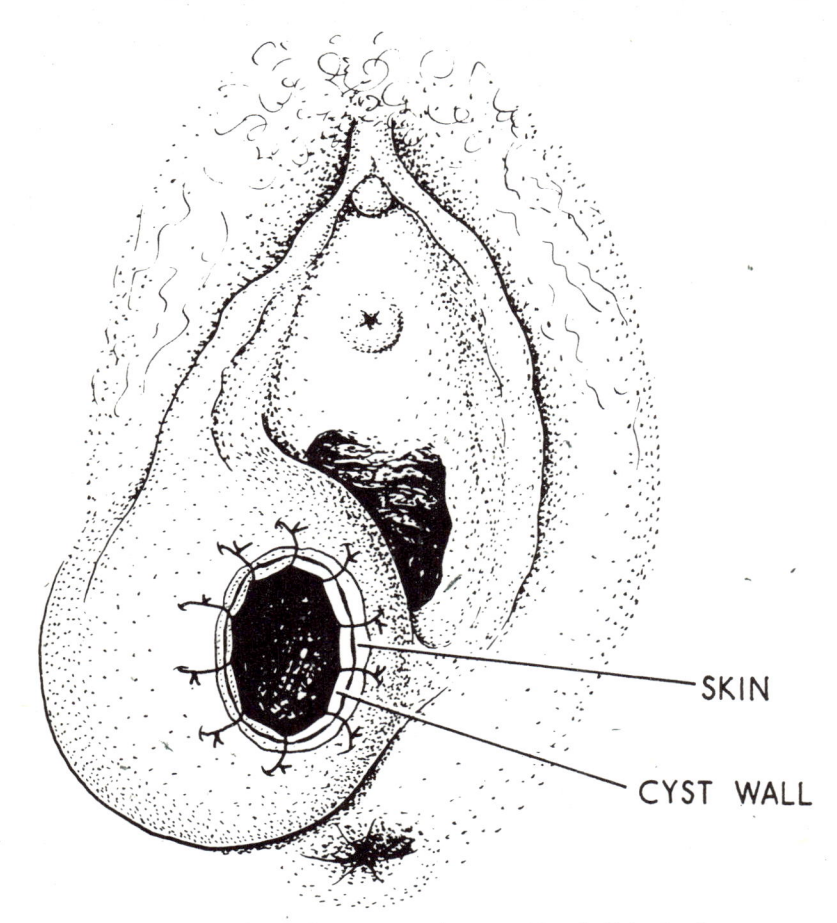

FIG. 67. Surgical treatment of a cyst of Bartholin's gland.

If it is left untreated the cyst will eventually burst or become infected. If it bursts it will slowly reform. The treatment is surgical by marsupialization of the cyst. A circle of skin whose size depends on the diameter of the cyst but is usually 2·5 cm. in diameter is excised over the cyst in the region of the hymen. An equal circle of the cyst wall is also excised and the raw edges of cyst wall and skin sutured with interrupted plan oo catgut. The patient may leave hospital in 1 or 2 days. No special post operative treatment is required other than twice daily baths. The sutures dissolve on the 4th and 5th day and do not therefore require removal. The end result is excellent; the cyst does not reform and the gland continues to function.

BARTHOLIN'S ABSCESS

This forms when a Bartholin cyst becomes infected. There is sudden onset of acute pain associated with a tender, red, œdematous swelling. Sitting and walking are most painful. The treatment is urgent marsupialization as for a Bartholin's cyst. A swab is taken for culture and the appropriate antibiotic given if required but usually the abscess settles rapidly and spontaneously when drained.

NEW GROWTHS OF THE VULVA

Carcinoma is the most common new growth of the vulva, and in many cases there is a history of leukoplakia or long-standing irritation. The growth first appears as a wart, nodule, hard fissure or ulcer. It is quite often bilateral, and may be found on the labia minora, clitoris or near the urethral orifice. Any such lesion in elderly women demands urgent biopsy.

The modern operation is a wide radical vulvectomy, which includes all the inguinal glands. The external iliac glands are also removed retroperitoneally by opening the abdomen as in an inguinal hernia operation. An extensive raw area is left which is not amenable to skin grafting, but must heal by granulation. The patient may be three months in hospital, and is a challenge to nursing skill and ingenuity.

A profuse serous discharge takes place from the raw areas, and it is very difficult to apply absorbent dressings to this region. Even if it were possible, such dressings would soon become painful as the discharge dried, and would predispose to infection. In the theatre after the operation a self-retaining catheter is inserted into the bladder, and tulle gras applied to the wound. Over this is placed a layer of skin muslin which is held in place by adhesive tape attaching the corners to normal skin. A blood transfusion is usually still in progress.

DISEASES OF THE VAGINA AND VULVA 149

A bed has been prepared for her in the ward with an air ring and a body cradle, and the attachments for the indwelling catheter are at the bedside. The patient is laid on her back, the catheter is connected to a uribag in the

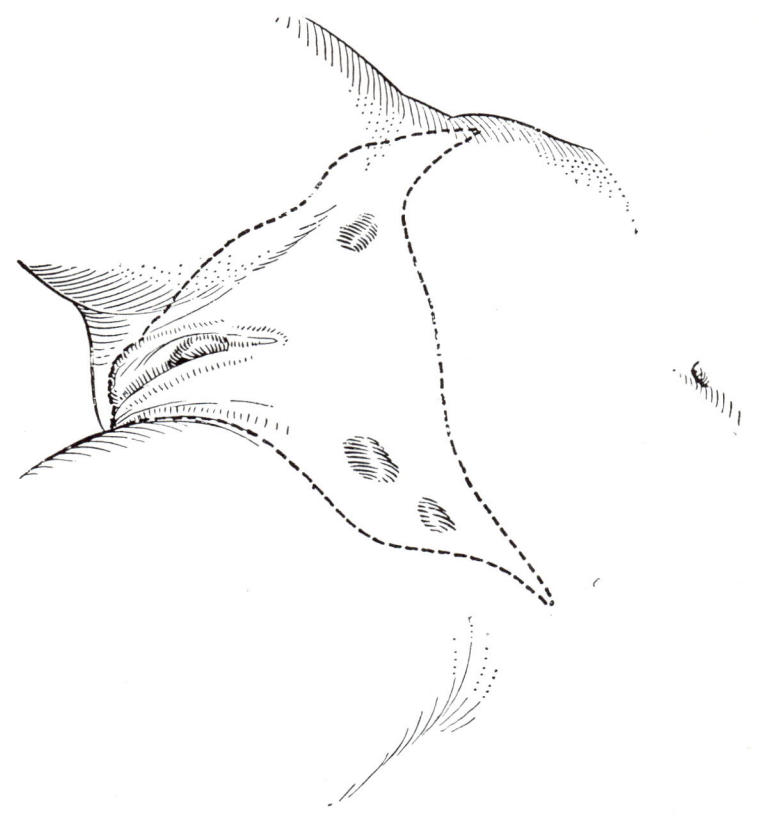

FIG. 68. The amount of tissue removed by radical vulvectomy. The shaded areas in the groins indicate glands to which spread may occur from a primary cancer of vulva.

theatre, a sterile pad put beneath the buttocks, and the cradle adjusted to keep the bedclothes from the operation area. When the required amount of blood has been given, dextran or glucose saline will be given by the intravenous route, and normally continue for forty-eight hours. A great deal of fluid is lost from the wound and it must be suitably replaced.

In view of the extensive raw operation site, the amount of pain felt is surprisingly small, and post-operative drugs in the usual amounts are sufficient. Fluids by mouth are given freely, and a diet with plenty of protein is prescribed, but high residue foods are omitted until the bowels have been opened on the fifth or sixth day. Drainage of the bladder is continued for about ten days.

The greatest problem will be the management of the wound. During the first day or two it will be necessary to renew the skin muslin at frequent intervals, often half-hourly, and clean drawsheets and ring covers will have to be supplied several times a day. The dressing must be done with all aseptic precautions to minimize infection, and the catheter must be cleaned, with glycerine or liquid paraffin swabs, of the encrusted discharge which rapidly collects. If possible, the tulle gras is not renewed until after the tenth day.

It is not possible to nurse the patient except on her back, so breathing exercises and leg movements are important to avert pneumonia and thrombosis.

Watch must also be kept on the character of the urine, since the catheter drainage may produce infection, unless the patient is given nitrofurantoin 100 mg. four times a day.

If infection becomes evident in the wound, a swab should be taken to identify the organism and its sensitivity, and antibiotics will often be necessary. On the twelfth day, the tulle gras should be removed if it has not had to be replaced earlier, and if possible the patient begins daily baths. From now on the dressings used depend on the state of the wound. Half strength eusol or $12\frac{1}{2}\%$ sodium sulphate, or red lotion, are good if there is infection; crude cod liver oil may be tried if granulation is slow. Care must be taken that the vaginal orifice is not sealed by granulation tissue at this stage. Ultra violet light and radiant heat both have their uses, and a warm current of air from an electric hair dryer four-hourly may help with moist patches.

This period is a very long tedious one for the patient and makes heavy demands of the nurse. In many cases, however, both have their reward since the outlook except in advanced disease is quite good. Healing takes place with much contracture (though this can be minimized by keeping

DISEASES OF THE VAGINA AND VULVA

the patient active), but with a reasonable prospect of cure.

VAGINAL DISCHARGE

The normal vaginal secretion consists of a transudation through the vaginal squamous epithelium in which there are no glands. The cervix and its glands supply a certain amount of mucous secretion and, at certain times in the menstrual cycle, glands of the endometrium also produce some secretion. During coitus, Bartholin's glands provide a lubricatory contribution. Normal vaginal secretion, therefore, consists of clear mucus from the cervix, clear watery-like transudation from the vaginal lining and epithelial debris from the vagina and uterus. This epithelial debris consists of the superficial squamous cells from the mucous membrane of the vagina. All women must have a little vaginal secretion to provide the necessary lubrication for this canal. The bowel and anal canal are similarly supplied. In some women, however, the amount is excessive and may be sufficient to be appreciated by the patient as a moistness around the vulva or on her underclothing. This excessive secretion is an exaggeration of the normal and will contain few pathogenic organisms and almost no pus cells. It, therefore, is not inflammatory in any way and should not be considered pathological. The discharge, strictly speaking, should only be considered abnormal or pathological if it is purulent, e.g., if, on microscopical examination, a large number of pus cells are present. In chronic discharges, however, although the pus cell content may be small, the amount lost may be considerable, e.g., in chronic cervicitis which has responded to treatment but where a clear excessive mucoid discharge persists. The term " leucorrhœa " means a white discharge and, unfortunately, is used quite inaccurately to mean any discharge of any nature or colour from the female genital tract.

A history is first taken. The patient's age, parity, menstrual habit and any associated symptoms are ascertained. The nature of the discharge, its quantity, the necessity for a pad, whether it is intermittent or continuous, offensive or not, are other important points. The patient's story and the gynæcologist's impression of the discharge are often quite dissimilar and some patients, especially young ones, may complain, perhaps because of a misdemeanour, real or imaginary, of a discharge which cannot be found.

The vulva is then inspected and the gynæcologist notes the nature of the discharge and its amount, whether the vulva is inflamed, whether the hymen is intact, and any local abnormality. A speculum examination is then made of the vagina and cervix, and material may be collected for bacteriological examination and a cervical and vaginal cytology smear taken. A wet film preparation is used in an examination for trichomonas and monilia. Gonorrhœa is excluded by means of a charcoal swab deposited in a small bottle of Stuart's transport medium after breaking off the end. If any urethral discharge is present, a swab must also be taken of this. Digital examination is then made of the uterus and appendages.

Leucorrhœa, or white discharge, may be found in a variety of conditions; it is sometimes associated with general diseases such as anæmia and rheumatoid arthritis. Bacteriological examination may need to be repeated to exclude infection.

A mucous discharge may be associated with an erosion of the cervix. A speculum examination shows a red area around the external os which is a downgrowth of the columnar epithelium of the cervical canal onto the vaginal portion of the cervix. A cervical polypus produces a similar discharge.

If the patient has had children, lacerations of the cervix which have become chronically infected may cause a mucopurulent discharge. One of the purposes of a post-natal examination is to treat such infections.

Offensive discharges may be associated with retained pessaries or other foreign bodies, trichomonas infection or carcinoma of the uterus. Fibroid polypi projecting into the vagina may ulcerate and cause the same symptom.

A slight blood-stained discharge is found in senile vaginitis but the first condition to exclude is carcinoma; a dilatation of the cervix and curettage of the uterus may therefore be indicated.

The treatment of a vaginal discharge is naturally that of the cause and is indicated under the appropriate sections. Erosion of the cervix can be treated by cautery if the discharge is sufficient to warrant it. Fibroid polypi must be

DISEASES OF THE VAGINA AND VULVA

cut or twisted from their attachment in the uterus and this should be done in the theatre, though small mucous polypi may be removed in the Out-patient Clinic. Chronic cervicitis is a loose term which embraces a torn cervix with an erosion and chronic infection in the glands of the endocervical canal. It undoubtedly gives rise to a mucous or mucopurulent discharge and a vague feeling of discomfort deep in the pelvis. The best treatment is diathermy conisation of the infected and involved parts of the cervix; the diathermy needle cuts away all the diseased area and leaves a charred scar in the base of a crater-shaped wound; this heals in about six weeks' time with surprisingly little deformity of the cervix. This has superseded the old operation of amputation of the cervix which is now very rarely performed. The results of conisation are excellent and it need not in any way interfere with future pregnancies. General conditions like anæmia should be treated and reassurance given to the worried patient.

Proprietary makes of tampon are on the market for use during menstruation and nurses are sometimes asked for their opinion on them. The answer is that they are not advisable for young girls who are not able to introduce them because the introitus is small; that they are often inadequate protection on the first day of the period when loss is free; obviously they must not be forgotten and left *in situ* until gross infection results. There is no medical objection to their use, and their social convenience is great.

VAGINAL FISTULÆ

A fistula is an abnormal communication between one organ and another, and those that occur in the vagina communicate either with the urinary system or with the rectum. The causes of fistulæ are:—

(*a*) Difficult deliveries, in which fistulæ may be caused by sloughing due to prolonged pressure, or to extensive tears of the perineum which have failed to heal completely.

(*b*) Injury to ureter or bladder during operation.

(*c*) Malignant disease involving bladder, ureter or rectum, as well as vagina.

(*d*) Radium injuries. The posterior vaginal wall and rectum are especially vulnerable to excessive radiation.

(e) Perforating injuries of the vagina, such as may be caused by criminal abortion.

Fistulæ are now much less common in this country than formerly because long difficult labours are more likely to be terminated by Cæsarean section, and because of improve-

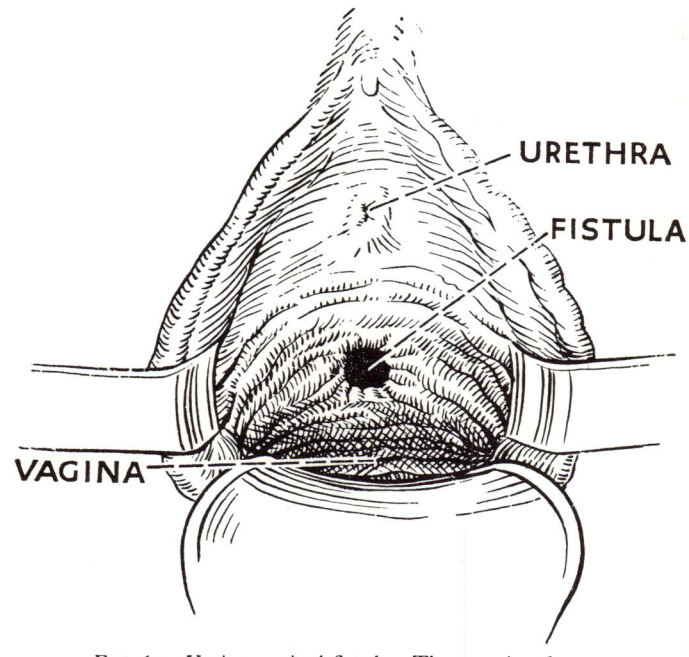

Fig. 69. Vesico-vaginal fistula. The opening from the vagina into the bladder is shown.

ments in the technique of irradiation. There are, however, many parts of the world where they are still common.

Urinary Fistulæ. The communication may be between bladder and vagina (VESICO-VAGINAL fistula) or between a ureter and the vagina (URETERO-VAGINAL). Urethro-vaginal fistulæ also occur, but much less commonly.

The patient with a urinary fistula complains of incontinence of urine, usually following a delivery or operation. It is important to decide whether it is the ureter or the bladder which is leaking into the vagina, and a careful history is taken, with especial regard to the amount lost, and whether normal micturition takes place as well. An examination of the vaginal walls is made, using a Sims'

DISEASES OF THE VAGINA AND VULVA

speculum, and the fistula sought. A catheter may be passed into the bladder, and indigo-carmine injected, and if the dye appears in the vagina, the fistula leads into the bladder, while if the urine appearing in the vagina remains clear it must be coming from the ureter. Cystoscopy is also necessary in order to inspect the fistula if it is a vesical one, or to determine which ureter is affected. In the latter case indigo-carmine is injected intravenously, and the efflux from the ureteric orifices watched through the cystoscope. If the fistula is a large one, cystoscopy may be impossible, because the bladder cannot be filled with fluid.

The patient's condition evokes sympathy, but operation must be delayed for six months from the time of onset in an obstetrical case. This allows the tissues to strengthen, inflammatory reaction to resolve and sepsis to be controlled. During this time the urine should be kept alkaline, and as the time for operation approaches, a catheter specimen of urine is examined for infection, and the blood urea estimated.

Several operations exist for the cure of vesico-vaginal fistulæ, all involving excision of the track and re-suture of the bladder and vagina. Continuous bladder drainage is employed, usually for fourteen days afterwards, and this is the most important point in post-operative care. The catheter may drain into a uribag or continuous suction may be used with a Robert's sucker to keep the bladder empty. In either case the nurse must assure herself by constant inspection that urine is draining continuously. If the catheter blocks and the bladder fills, the bladder wound may reopen and the fistula be re-established. The patient will have to undergo a further period of waiting, in much physical misery, for a second operation, which is naturally more difficult to perform than the first.

After fourteen days the catheter is removed, and normal micturition encouraged. Retention of urine must be prevented by the utmost vigilance on the part of the nurse. Even if micturition appears satisfactory, it is best to pass a catheter daily until residual urine does not exceed 100 ml. (3 oz.).

Damage to a ureter at operation should be detected by the surgeon, and dealt with in the way described on p. 54.

RECTO-VAGINAL FISTULA

A recto-vaginal fistula usually opens into the middle third of the vagina, and if it is large enough, will allow fæces as well as flatus to pass into the vagina. Carcinoma of cervix may create such a fistula, but in a patient in the late stages of malignant disease treatment can only be directed towards minimizing discomfort. Radiation burns are very rarely seen now, but when seen tend to be extensive, often necessitating a colostomy before treatment is undertaken.

The fistula most amenable to treatment is that following extensive tears during childbirth. Precipitate or unassisted labour may result in a tear extending through the vagina and perineum into the rectum, i.e., a complete or third degree tear. Complete tears are most often seen in patients with an android or masculine type of pelvis, in which there is little room in the fore pelvis. Such an injury is not common nowadays, especially since the practice of episiotomy

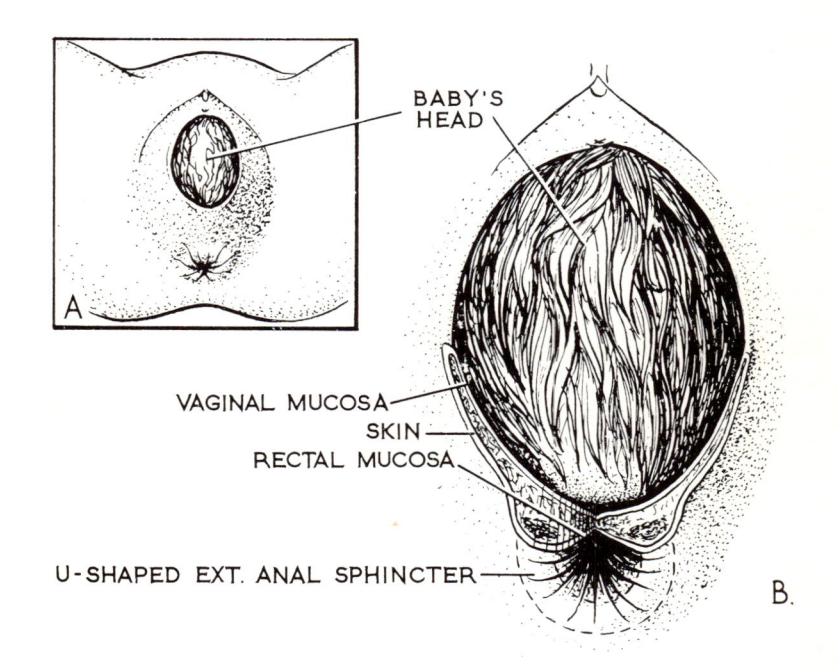

FIG. 70. A. The perineum is thinned by the advancing head.
B. In unfavourable circumstances the perineum may split, even into the rectum.

DISEASES OF THE VAGINA AND VULVA

(*q.v.*) to enlarge the vaginal outlet if a tear seemed imminent has become widespread.

All tears are carefully and accurately sutured in a good light. If a complete tear occurs in a case being delivered in her own home, she would be admitted to hospital for repair under good conditions with regard to light, anæsthesia and asepsis. Following suture the bowels are kept confined for three days, vitamin C is given to promote healing, and steps are taken to deal with any local infection. Should the wound unite at its lower end, but fail to heal completely in its upper part, a recto-vaginal fistula results.

Operation for repair is undertaken six months later and a good result is usually obtained. The large intestine must be quite empty before operation, and a course of phthalyl sulphathiazole can be given for five days, G. 2 four-hourly, to sterilize the bowel. Vitamin K should also be given, since vitamin formation by the intestinal bacteria will have been halted by the drug and bleeding may result after operation, due to a fall in the prothrombin level in the blood.

After the fistula has been repaired, the patient is given a low residue diet and the bowels confined for five days, and easy action should finally be obtained with the aid of liquid paraffin by mouth and olive oil per rectum. All straining must be avoided until the vaginal wound is soundly healed, and if ever a vaginal discharge indicates infection, a swab is taken and chemotherapy should be begun.

Very occasionally a recto-vaginal fistula may follow a posterior colpo-perineorrhaphy for prolapse, if the rectum has injured at operation.

CHAPTER 9

SEXUALLY TRANSMITTED DISEASES

The number of diseases and infestations that can be passed from one person to another during sexual activity runs into double figures, and of these three are defined, in the legal sense, as venereal diseases; these are syphilis, gonorrhœa, and chancroid. The last is relatively uncommon outside the tropics; syphilis, the most dangerous of the three, is still increasing in developing countries but elsewhere its advance is slowing; the figures for gonorrhœa are rising everywhere in the world, and in some places it is the commonest infectious disease. Effective treatment exists for all the sexually transmitted diseases, and yet a

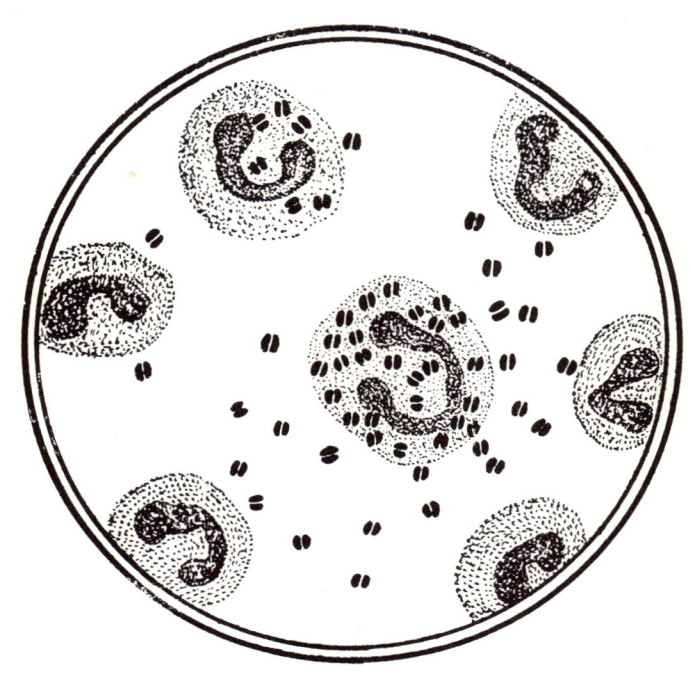

FIG. 71. Gonococci. The large objects shown are pus cells. Among them and within them are the gonococci seen in pairs.

VENEREAL DISEASE

mounting number of people are infected. It is important to consider not only the course and treatment of these diseases, but also the social causes and possible means of control of these conditions, which can cause so much personal stress and anxiety, and in some cases crippling ill health.

GONORRHŒA

Gonorrhœa is caused by the gonococcus, an organism which infects primarily the mucous membrane of the genital tract in both sexes. The incubation period is generally from three to ten days, but may be as long as three weeks. In men, the symptoms of burning pain on micturition and purulent urethral discharge are so well marked that early treatment is usually sought. In women, however, the course is different. 80% of women have no symptoms at all, which means that they remain infectious to others, and that complications are relatively more common than in men. Pain and frequency of micturition may be ascribed to cystitis, and though purulent vaginal discharge from the

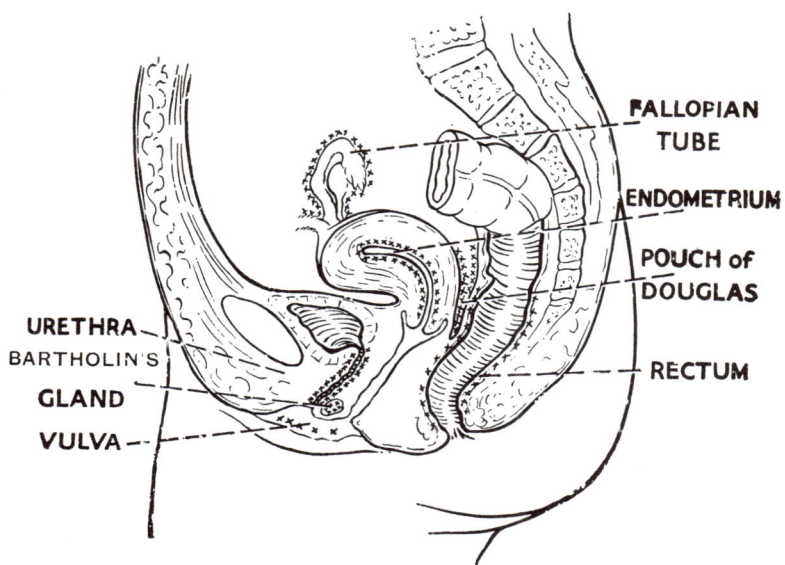

FIG. 72. Possible sites of spread of acute gonorrhœa. Inflammation of the urethra, cervix, and vulva is usual. Spread to the endometrium, Fallopian tubes, peritoneal cavity, and also to the rectum can occur.

infected cervix may occur, it is often so slight as to pass unnoticed. The vulva may be red and inflamed, and sometimes Bartholin's glands may be infected. Rectal infection (proctitis) occasionally occurs, but the most important complication is the spread of infection to the Fallopian tubes. About five hundred women contract salpingitis (p. 84) every year in this country, and of these the majority will become sterile, because adhesions of the complex folds of the mucous membrane of the tubes prevents the passage of egg cells from the ovaries to the uterus.

If a baby is born to a woman with gonorrhœa, its eyes may become infected during its passage through the birth canal, and the resulting infection, ophthalmia neonatorum may, if not successfully treated, result in loss of sight. Up to very recent times, ophthalmia was the main cause of congenital blindness. The decline in this disease is due to these causes:—

(1) Efficient antenatal care and early diagnosis.
(2) Effective treatment is now available.
(3) Care is taken at the birth of the baby to wipe its lids with a swab, if possible before the eyes are open. Any discharge from the eyes in the newly born child is reported by the midwife to a doctor.

Treatment of gonorrhoea is by penicillin. The large majority of patients can be cured by a single injection, though the dose has risen over the years as the gonococcus shows increasing resistance to penicillin. Highly resistant strains can be treated by other antibiotics, and these can also be used if the patient is allergic to penicillin. Bacteriological confirmation or cure is necessary before the patient can be pronounced free from infection.

A special form of gonorrhœa, not acquired venereally, occasionally spreads in communities of small girls, and causes vulvo-vaginitis. The lining of the adult vagina is resistant to infection, but children before puberty are very susceptible. The condition is treated by penicillin, and sometimes small doses of stilbœstrol sufficient to produce an acid reaction in the vagina. Hygienic precautions with clothes, towels and lavatory seats must be taken to prevent further spread.

The complication of gonorrhœa most likely to be seen

by the gynæcologist is salpingitis. The patient may present with an acute infection, or with the chronic inflammatory sequel, or may be met in the infertility clinic, since even a mild attack of salpingitis may cause adhesions of its ciliated lining which form a barrier to the passage of the ovum.

NON-SPECIFIC URETHRITIS

Urethritis in men is in many cases not gonococcal in origin, and because no infecting organism has been identified, this condition is termed non-specific or non-gonococcal urethritis. Since figures began to be recorded separately from gonorrhoea in 1951, the known incidence has steadily risen. No corresponding condition has been identified in women, but there is no doubt that it is a sexually transmitted disease. In a few men, arthritis, iritis and skin lesions can occur (constituting Reiter's syndrome), and prolonged ill health results. Since the cause is unknown, treatment is less than satisfactory, but antibiotics are used.

SYPHILIS

Syphilis has been known in Europe since the end of the fifteenth century, and while never as common as gonorrhœa is more destructive in its effects. The cause is the treponema pallidum (spirochæta pallida) and it may be acquired as the result of intercourse with a contagious person, or appear in congenital form in children of a syphilitic mother. The disease runs a long course, and the clinical picture changes markedly from one stage to the next.

ACQUIRED SYPHILIS

Early Infectious Syphilis. About four weeks after infection (in most cases nine to ninety days) an ulcer appears at the site of infection, usually on the vulva but sometimes on the cervix where it may be unnoticed. This is the primary or hard sore, and the serum that oozes from the floor of the ulcer is contagious. The glands in the groin are usually swollen but not tender, and general symptoms are absent. Even if untreated the ulcer heals in a month or two.

From six to eight weeks after the appearance of the primary sore the general signs and symptoms of the secondary stage manifest themselves. There is a slight rise in the temperature, headache, anæmia, lassitude, lymph-

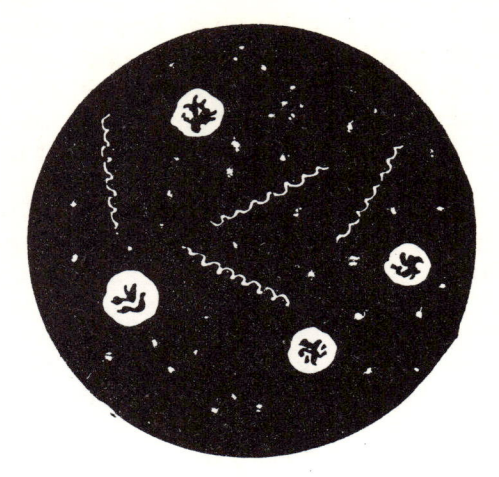

FIG. 73. Spirochætes. The corkscrew shape is characteristic; pus cells are also shown.

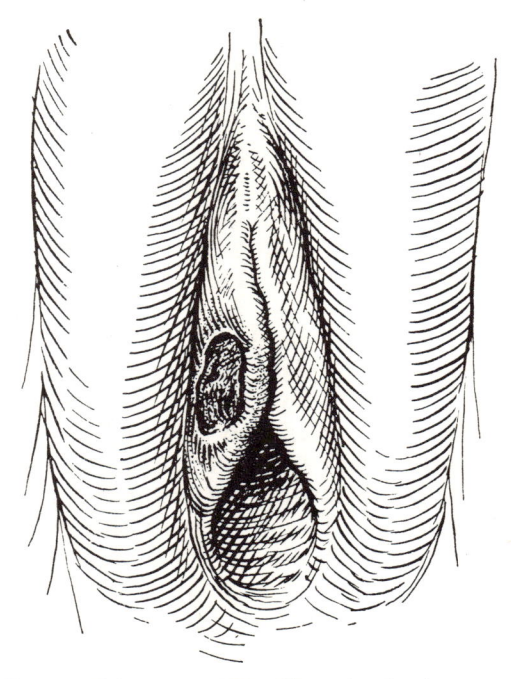

FIG 74. Primary Syphilis. There is a hard sore on the right labium minus.

VENEREAL DISEASE

adenitis, and hoarseness and sore throat due to ulceration of the fauces. Around the anus and spreading on to the vulva appear sodden masses of heaped up epithelium called

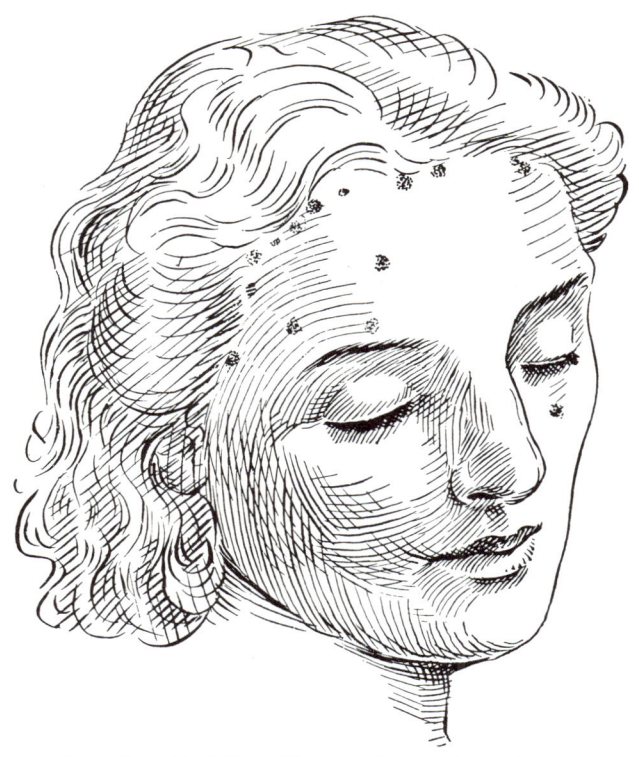

FIG. 75. Secondary Syphilis. The maculo-papular rash often appears on the face, or may typically be seen as shown along the hair margin. ("corona veneris.")

condylomata lata. Rashes of many kinds appear on the face, trunk and limbs; they are symmetrical, non-irritating and often of a brownish-red colour. The reaction of the serum to the Wassermann and similar tests is always positive, and the moist lesions are very contagious.

These signs and symptoms too may disappear without treatment, though often with recurrences and the patient passes into a latent stage, where signs are absent, but reactivity of the disease process is always possible.

Late Syphilis. After two years the lesions of syphilis are non-contagious, and there may be several further years of latency before other signs appear. The characteristic lesion of the third or tertiary stage is the gumma, which is an inflammatory zone surrounding an area of necrosis and forming a lump, which if near the surface breaks down to form a chronic ulcer. These lesions may affect skin, subcutaneous tissues, mucous membrane, bones or viscera. Later still such diseases as general paralysis of the insane, tabes dorsalis, syphilitic aneurysm and disease of the aortic valves are examples of the late effects of syphilis on the nervous and cardio-vascular systems. On these a textbook of medicine should be consulted.

Congenital Syphilis

One of the tragic aspects of syphilis is that it appears in a congenital form in the babies of infected mothers. Within a few weeks of birth the baby begins to lose weight, has nasal discharge and sores at the angles of the mouth. A brownish-red rash appears, which when on the buttocks must be differentiated from a napkin rash. All these early lesions are infectious. The later stigmata include the saddle nose caused by collapse of the nasal bones due to ulceration, scars (rhagades) at the corners of the mouth, notching of the central incisors of the permanent teeth (Hutchinson's teeth) and haziness of the cornea due to interstitial keratitis. Gummatous lesions like those of the adult may also appear.

Successful antenatal care can prevent this infection. All pregnant women should have a serological test for syphilis, and if this is positive energetic treatment is undertaken, which may be repeated for subsequent pregnancies.

Serological Tests

The best known test is the Wassermann, while the Kahn and Price precipitation reaction are also widely used. These tests do not demonstrate the presence of a specific antibody to syphilis in the blood, and occasionally a false positive reaction may be displayed by those who have had certain tropical and virus infections. The treponema pallidum immobilization (T.P.I.) test of Nelson is used to eliminate these.

VENEREAL DISEASE

TREATMENT

Congenital. Penicillin (e.g. 400,000 units per kg. body weight given over a period of ten days) is effective. The general medical and nursing care of an ill baby are the same as those given to the marasmic babies.

Acquired. For the early case, penicillin followed by a course of intramuscular injections of bismuth is given. For the late manifestations, this treatment is preceded by a preliminary course of bismuth. The older anti-syphilitic drugs, such as the arsenicals, are not now used.

OTHER SEXUALLY TRANSMITTED CONDITIONS

Thrush (p. 140) and trichomonas infection, (p. 139) can produce symptoms in men as well as women. Scabies can be contracted by sharing a bed with an infected partner, and infestation by crab lice is readily passed on. Genital warts are very commonly seen in venereal disease clinics; like warts elsewhere in the skin, they result from virus infection. Another virus condition is herpes genitalis, similar to but not identical with that causing the cold sores that often occur on the lips. These may seem minor in comparison with syphilis and gonorrhoea, but they are depressing and sometimes painful, and cause much personal misery and stress, while those which produce breaks in the skin and mucous membrane can open up channels by which more serious infection can enter.

CONTROL OF VENEREAL INFECTION

Variations in economic development, style of living both urban and rural, and adequacy of medical services means that venereal disease problems differ in all parts of the world, but everywhere the incidence of these diseases is rising. In this country, the method of attack is to provide free and confidential advice and treatment to all who will avail themselves; to seek to trace contacts and persuade them to accept treatment, and to publicize the subject through the mass media such as radio, television and the press. There are one or two hopeful signs; syphilis, for instance, seems to be coming under control, because the long incubation period favours the tracing and effective treatment of contacts. Efficient antenatal care has made congenital syphilis uncommon, and the long-term complications of syphilis are now becoming rare. Gonococcal ophthalmia is now rarely seen because it is prevented by the vigilance of midwives and obstetricians.

The position however with regard to gonorrhoea is very disturbing. There is no sign that the rising incidence is levelling off, and an increasing number of young and very young people are affected. Twenty years ago, infected men outnumbered women by four to one, but now the sex ratio among the young is almost equal. Various reasons are suggested for this; one is the increasing popularity as a means of contraception of the pill, which provides no protection against infection as the sheath did. Another is that women tend to expect as one aspect of emancipation that they may adopt the same standards of sexual behaviour that men do.

Some reasons for the increase in venereal infection are outside our control; for instance, the population of the world is increasing, and the age of reaching sexual capability is falling, so that there is a greater number of people at risk, and the length of their active sexual life is increasing. It has long been known that wars were associated with a rise in venereal disease because large numbers of men were uprooted from their own home life and lived in conditions of tension and anxiety alternating with boredom. There are still many men serving overseas all over the world, and in addition there has never been a time of greater social upheaval than exists today. People are everywhere moving from rural areas into cities, or from one country to another in search of work or a better life, holiday makers travel the world, and everywhere settled patterns of life are being disrupted.

In addition, the present public attitude to sex has been much modified in recent times. Sex is now openly discussed, and so receives increasing attention from films, the press, radio and television. Since all behaviour is learned, the constant pressure of commercial advertising and the mass media may lead young people to think of promiscuity as normal, while their parents may be dismayed and confused at the state of the world as they see it, and not feel confident enough to offer advice or defend principles which the young may deride as old fashioned.

"Education" is often advocated, and it is important

VENEREAL DISEASE

that factual information rather than vague precepts should be given to young people. They should know that intercourse may result not only in unwanted pregnancy but in infection; that the pill may protect against pregnancy but not against venereal disease; that those who change partners frequently or affairs with chance acquaintances stand a very high chance of getting one of the sexually transmitted conditions; that one attack of gonorrhœa gives no immunity to further attacks; and that free advice and treatment is available.

Prevention is obviously better than cure, even though there is a cure, and avoidance of exposure to infection is the best prevention. Work is in progress on the possibility of immunization against gonorrhœa, but the fact that people can get repeated attacks is not a hopeful sign. No one should however accept that a high level of sexually transmitted disease is inevitable in our present social climate, and we can seek to show the advantages of a more stable attitude to sex, both to the individual and the community.

CHAPTER 10
PROBLEMS OF FERTILITY

" INFERTILITY " is a better word than " sterility " since the latter, when applied to a married couple, means that there is no possibility of pregnancy. The psychological impact of being told that one or other partner can never produce a child may be sufficient to break up the marriage or, at least, precipitate a serious matrimonial crisis. A young married couple should not consider themselves infertile until at least two years have elapsed after marriage. If, however, a woman marries later in life—in, say the late thirties—it is important not to allow so long an interval before starting investigations.

Although a woman will usually present herself and will usually regard herself as responsible for the infertility, the husband is, in fact, responsible in about one-third of all cases and he should, therefore, be investigated as well as the wife. The best procedure is for the husband to be examined by a doctor who specializes in male infertility and this examination will include a full general examination of the patient and examination of his genital system. This may reveal, for example, absence or maldescent of the testicles or, perhaps, some developmental abnormality of the male organ, e.g., hypospadias. If, however, the man is found on clinical examination to be normal, a special examination should be made of his semen; each millilitre of this should contain one hundred million live and active spermatozoa. Although it only takes one spermatozoon to fertilize an ovum, it is a surprising finding that men with less than forty million spermatozoa per millilitre are relatively infertile.

Having established that the husband is satisfactory, the investigation of the wife should now be undertaken. It is assumed, in the first instance, that she is clinically normal and that her general constitutional and endocrine make-up is normal; also, that a bimanual pelvic examination shows that her uterus is normal in size, position and consistence, with normal appendages. Two special investigations must now be undertaken:—

(1) It must be established that the tubes are patent and function normally; this is done by passing a small quantity of carbon dioxide gas via a cannula in the cervix, through the uterus and along the tubes so that it escapes into the peritoneal cavity. The gas collects under the diaphragm which it irritates and produces a reflex pain in the patient's shoulder, which is diagnostic of tubal patency. In addition, the behaviour of the recording pen on the revolving drum of the tubal patency apparatus will also show if the tube is patent. It is important to test the tubal patency immediately after a period as, at this time, the tubal mucous membrane is not congested and false readings will not occur. Just before menstruation, however, the mucous membrane is congested and it is possible to rupture a small vessel and inject the gas directly into the vein; with carbon dioxide, which is the proper gas to use, there is no danger but, if atmospheric air is used, the danger of an air embolism from nitrogen bubbles is considerable and, in fact, there have been a number of reported fatalities. Some surgeons employ radio-opaque substances which they inject up a cannula into the uterus and tubes which are then outlined and can be seen under the X-ray screen; this second method demonstrates the site of any obstruction in the tube, and also its exact shape and size.

(2) If the tubes have been proved to be patent and gas passes at the normal pressure of about 60 mm., the woman is next investigated to determine whether she is ovulating or not. Some women menstruate quite regularly but they have anovular cycles and, without an ovum, fertilization cannot occur. Moreover, if there is no ovum, there is no Graafian follicle to rupture and, therefore, no corpus luteum will be formed in the ovary; if there is no corpus luteum, there will be no progesterone produced and, therefore, no progestational changes in the endometrium in the premenstrual phase. A biopsy of the endometrium a day or so before the expected date of menstruation should therefore be performed and the specimen, prepared as a microscopic slide, will immediately show whether there are progestational changes or not; if not, the woman is not ovulating. It must be remembered, however, that women

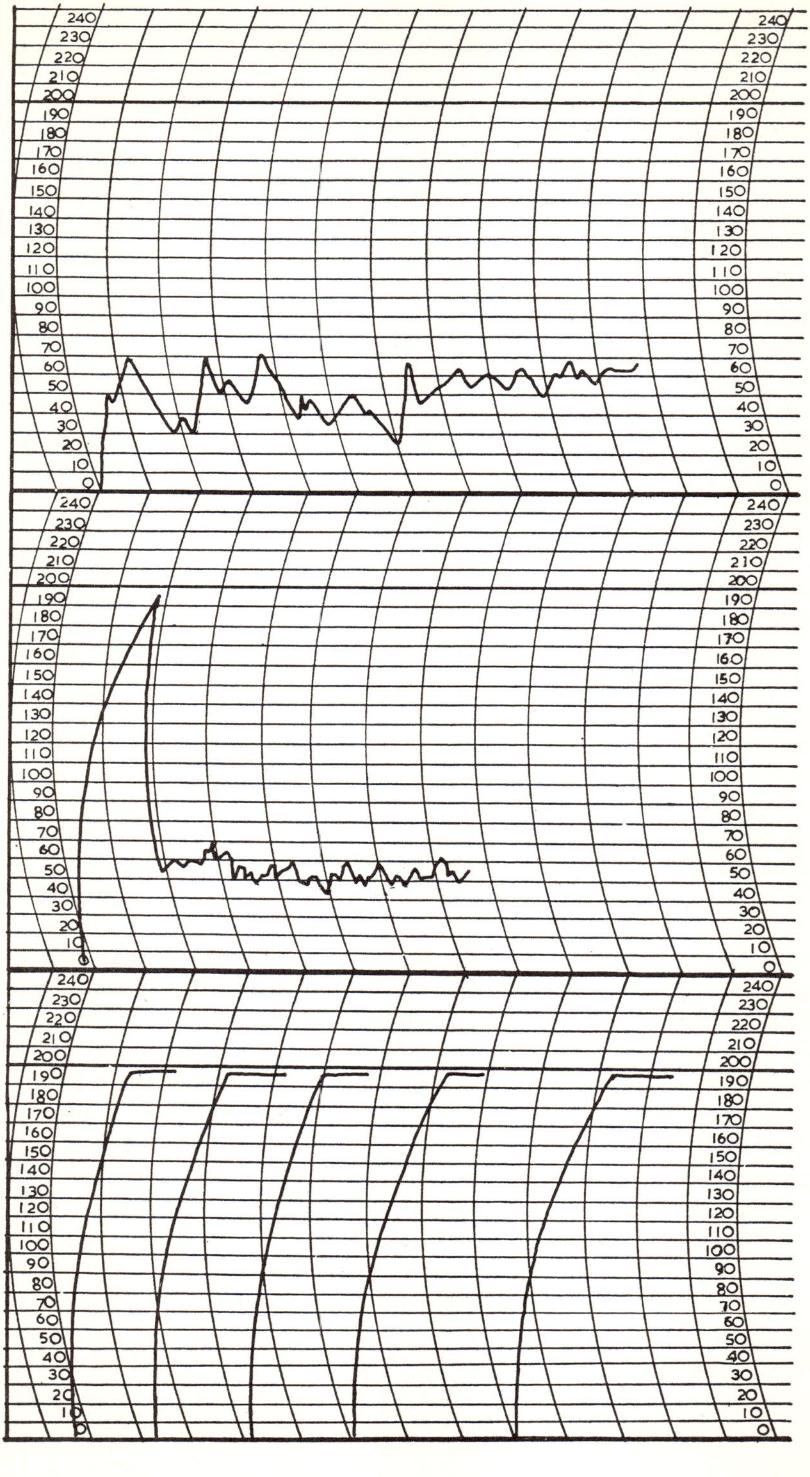

240
230
220
210
200
190
180
170
160
150
140
130
120
110
100
90
80
70
60
50
40
30
20
10
0

A

B

C

are not bound by any law of physiology and that they may have an anovular menstrual cycle one month and an ovular cycle the next, so that the finding of an anovular cycle on one occasion does not necessarily indicate permanent infertility.

There are other methods of determining whether a woman is ovulating or not but none so satisfactory as a biopsy. One of these consists of instructing her to take her morning temperature and to prepare a chart; during the pre-ovulatory phase, her temperature is about 0·5 to 1° C. lower than after she has ovulated and this so-called biphasic reaction is strongly suggestive that a woman has ovulated. A further method of determining whether ovulation has occurred is the estimation of the end-product of progesterone metabolism in the urine; this substance is called pregnanediol; the method, however, is elaborate, time-consuming and expensive. Examination of vaginal smears will also show if ovulation has occurred.

Let us now assume that we have established the satisfactory capabilities of the husband and that the wife has a normal pelvis on clinical examination, patent tubes and that she is ovulating regularly. Such a couple should be reassured and encouraged to be optimistic about the future. There is no doubt that a state of anxiety neurosis can be engendered in one or both parties of an infertile marriage which has a deleterious effect on impregnation and many cases are recorded where an infertile couple has been encouraged to adopt a baby; as soon as they have done this and ceased to worry about their own fertility, conception very promptly occurs. It is assumed from this that over-anxiety on the part of the wife can cause spasm of some part of the genital tract, probably the tube, thereby rendering it impervious. It is fair to state that, whether this spasm theory is correct or not, there are many obscure factors operating in an infertile marriage. One of these which has

FIG. 76. Kymographs.
- (*A*) Normal kymograph. At a pressure of 60 mm. of mercury, gas passes from the tubes into the peritoneal cavity.
- (*B*) Spasm of the tubes. A pressure of 195 mm. is necessary before the gas enters the peritoneal cavity.
- (*C*) Occlusion of the tubes. The pressure has been raised five times to 195 mm., but without avail.

never been proved, is the theory of biological incompatibility in which A marries B and the marriage is infertile and dissolved; A then marries C and B then marries D and both of these couples now produce children.

In this section on infertility, it has been assumed that the woman is completely normal on pelvic examination and that all such abnormalities as excessive vaginal discharge or erosion of the cervix have been corrected before any investigation is undertaken. Similarly, any fibroids which are present in the uterus should be removed by the operation of myomectomy. Although these minor abnormalities may not in themselves constitute a bar to conception and many women with a gross vaginal discharge and unhealthy cervices readily conceive, in an infertile marriage it is important to correct every possible abnormality, however minor.

CONTROL OF CONCEPTION

In modern society many married couples wish to control not only the number of children in their family but also the timing of the arrival of their children. There are many methods whereby a couple can live a normal married life and yet plan their family with a certain degree of accuracy. The method selected must accord with the religious beliefs of the couple, their economic and living conditions, and the acceptability of the means to them from the æsthetic point of view.

These may be broadly classified as follows:—

(1) The restriction of sexual intercourse
    (*a*) Abstinence for several months or even years.
    (*b*) Abstinence during the fertile phase of the menstrual cycle.

(2) Methods to prevent conception used by the female
    (*a*) The insertion of spermicidal substances in the vagina.
    (*b*) The use of an occlusive diaphragm placed in the vagina to prevent the sperms gaining access to the cervical canal.
    (*c*) Altering the consistency of the cervical mucus so that the sperms are killed.
    (*d*) Placing a device within the uterine cavity.

PROBLEMS OF FERTILITY

(e) Suppressing ovulation.

(3) Methods available to the male
  (a) Coitus interruptus.
  (b) The use of a sheath or condom to prevent the escape of sperms into the vagina.
  (c) The suppression of the formation of sperms by hormones or chemicals.

(1) Restriction of intercourse
(a) **Abstinence for several months or even years.**
Total abstinence may be practised by some people for months or even years, but this is not usually acceptable as a method of conception control. It is sometimes practised by married couples who have a large family and who have been too embarrassed to seek proper advice on the problem of control of conception. It is worth pointing out at this stage that the spermatozoa deposited at the vaginal entrance can be capable of migrating up the vagina and thus resulting in pregnancy.

(b) **Abstinence during the fertile phase of the menstrual cycle.**
This is a widely practised method of the control of conception and is based on the principle that ovulation occurs 14 days before the next menstrual period. In a 28 day menstrual cycle therefore ovulation occurs on day 14. The ovum probably lives for only 12 or 18 hours. The spermatozoa however will remain alive in the female genital tract for up to three days. If the first day of the menstrual period is counted as day one of the menstrual cycle then pregnancy may occur if intercourse takes place on the 11th, 12th, 13th or 14th day. Thus it is between day 11 and day 14 that conception is most likely to occur. Although ovulation usually occurs on the 14th day of a 28 day cycle, some minor irregularities in the timing of ovulation may occur so that the egg may be formed at any stage from the 11th day to the 17th day. In order therefore to be absolutely safe intercourse should be avoided from the 9th to the 17th day. From this it can be seen that pregnancy is unlikely to occur if intercourse takes place between the 1st and the 8th day or between the 18th and 28th day of the menstrual cycle and these are therefore known as the safe periods of the cycle. This type of conception control is also known as the **rhythm method.**

The main difficulty with the rhythm method of conception control occurs when a person has an irregular menstrual cycle so that the date of ovulation cannot be predicted with any accuracy. Any woman however who has a regular menstrual cycle can work out the safe periods once she appreciates that ovulation occurs 14 days prior to the next menstrual period. Conception may occur on the estimated date of ovulation or on upon five days before and three days after that date.

The efficacy of this method of control of conception depends upon the regularity of the menstrual cycle together with the intellect of the couple and their ability to stick to the rules. Even so, spurious or irregular ovulation may occasionally occur, and pregnancy ensue even if the rules have been rigidly followed.

(2) Methods used by the female

(a) **The insertion of spermicidal substances in the vagina.**

There are many highly efficient and completely innocuous spermicidal agents which can be placed in the vagina and which will kill the spermatozoa very rapidly. A soluble pessary may be placed in the top of the vagina a short time before intercourse takes place. The pessary melts at body temperature and sperms deposited in the vagina are rapidly killed.

Tampons or sponges containing a spermicidal solution may be placed in the top of the vagina. These act not only by killing the sperms but also by hindering or preventing their access to the cervical canal.

The use of spermicidal pessaries and tampons is regarded as a very inefficient method of conception control.

(b) **The use of an occlusive diaphragm placed in the vagina to prevent the sperms gaining access to the cervical canal.**

Two main types of occlusive diaphragm may be used. The cervical cap is a dome shaped cap made of fairly thick plastic measuring approximately three centimetres in diameter and which fits accurately over the cervix.

The vaginal diaphragm or Dutch cap is a larger occlusive diaphragm which is placed in the vagina. It is made of thin rubber or plastic with a small spring welded into its circular edge and measures between six to nine centimetres in diameter.

Occlusive diaphragms prevent spermatozoa gaining access to the cervical canal. They should be combined with the use of a spermicidal cream or jelly. They are a fairly efficient method of conception control and third only to suppression of ovulation and the intrauterine device. They are acceptable to many women and are extensively used.

(c) **Altering the consistency of the cervical mucus so that the sperms are killed.**

Vaginal acidity kills spermatozoa fairly rapidly and any spermatozoa which are to survive and certainly any that are to fertilize an ovum must gain rapid access to the cervical canal. The cervical mucus is alkaline and is a medium in which spermatozoa can survive for relatively long periods. Any change in the alkalinity or the chemical composition of cervical mucus may render it lethal to spermatozoa. It is very probable that conception control in the future may be designed to alter cervical mucus in such a way that it becomes an inpenetrable barrier to spermatozoa.

(d) **Placing a device within the uterine cavity.**

Intrauterine contraceptive devices have been used for many years. The modern devices are made from metal or plastic and are inserted into the cavity of the uterus either with or without anæsthesia. They are made in various shapes, of which rings, coils and spirals are the most popular. Some of the plastic devices have thin nylon threads which protrude downwards through the cervical canal and can be palpated in the upper part of the vagina so that after insertion the patient can examine herself at frequent intervals (usually after a menstrual period) to reassure herself that the device is still in situ.

Intrauterine contraceptive devices are increasing in popularity because they are a very efficient method of conception control. Their exact mode of action is unknown but it is thought that it is effected by bringing about several changes in the female genital tract such as alteration in the cervical mucus; alteration in the intrauterine environment; increasing peristalsis in the Fallopian tubes so that the fertilized ovum reaches the uterus before it is ready to embed, **or** by preventing the fertilized ovum from embedding in the endometrium when it reaches the uterus at the normal times.

These devices occasionally cause side effects which render them unacceptable to the patient. They may cause menorrhagia, intermenstrual bleeding, vaginal discharge or dysmenorrhœa. Prolongation of the menstrual flow is usual for the first two or three cycles after their insertion, but this usually subsides and the periods return almost to normal, although most patients admit that the periods are slightly longer and heavier when a device is in situ.

(e) **Suppressing ovulation.**

Suppression of ovulation by the "pill" is now a well known method of conception control. The pill contains hormones which exert an action on either the ovary or the pituitary and thereby suppress ovulation. They are usually taken for 20 or 21 days in each menstrual cycle starting on the 5th day of the menstrual period.

These oral contraceptives, of which there are many available, are undoubtedly the most efficient method of conception control. They do however have advantages as well as disadvantages. In favour of oral contraceptives is their undoubted efficiency, together with the fact that they regulate the menstrual cycle to 28 days and reduce the quantity and duration of the loss. Among their disadvantages are the facts that they may cause weight gain, together with symptoms of irritability and headache due to fluid retention. They are contraindicated in certain conditions such as liver disease and cancer as well as in any patient who has previously suffered from any thromboembolic phenomenon. Their association with blood clotting is not definitely established but they do seem to influence the blood clotting mechanism and there is increasing evidence that they predispose certain patients to pulmonary embolus. They are also contraindicated in some types of cardiac and mental disease but there is no evidence that they cause cancer of the uterus.

(3) Methods used by Men

(a) **Coitus interruptus.**

Withdrawal of the male immediately prior to ejaculation is a widely practised method of conception control. It is highly inefficient and may be psychologically harmful to both partners. It is inefficient because secretions from the prostate which occur during intercourse may contain spermatozoa even prior to actual ejaculation.

(*b*) **The use of a sheath or condom to prevent the escape of sperms into the vagina.**

The use of a condom or sheath by the male is also a widely practised method of conception control. It is not as efficient as the oral contraceptives, the intrauterine devices or the vaginal diaphragm but has nevertheless been widely practised very successfully for many years.

(*c*) **The suppression of the formation of sperms by hormones or chemicals.**

The theoretical possibility of oral contraception for the male has been considered for many years. Drugs are known which will suppress spermatogenesis in the male and would be satisfactory male oral contraceptives but the drugs which have so far been experimentally produced have very severe side effects which render them unsuitable.

CHAPTER 11

GYNÆCOLOGICAL OPERATIONS

The management of a gynæcological theatre does not differ in any material respect from that of any other. The amount of emergency work tends to be smaller than in the general theatre, unless the hospital is in the kind of residential area which provides a number of incomplete abortions. There will be cases of twisted ovarian cysts and emergency Cæsarean sections, but most of the work will be on patients with severe bleeding like those mentioned above.

The instruments are, of course, special to the theatre, and the stock of drugs carried will include ergometrine, syntocinon and pitocin, which are oxytocics, or drugs which contract the uterus, and lobeline and nalorphine to stimulate respiration in the baby. Amyl nitrite capsules are also useful, since their inhalation may relax contraction rings in the uterus, or spasm in the Fallopian tubes.

Since operations are either abdominal or vaginal or both in approach, it is convenient for the theatre staff to have a foundation set for use in either case, and to add to it the extra instruments used for any particular operation. The types of forceps and needle holders used will vary greatly, but the lists given here indicate the sort of instruments needed.

A sterile catheter trolley should always be kept laid in the anæsthetic room on operating days, and on the bottom of the trolley should be sponge-holding forceps and receiver for removing pads or vaginal packs from the anæsthetized patient before she enters the theatre.

ABDOMINAL FOUNDATION SET

2 Bard Parker handles and blades of the surgeon's choice.
2 pairs of toothed dissecting forceps.
2 pairs of plain dissecting forceps.
1 pair of $7\frac{1}{2}$ in. dissecting forceps.
1 pair of plain forceps for sister's needles.
2 pairs of curved Mayo scissors, large.
2 pairs of surgeon's straight scissors.

GYNÆCOLOGICAL OPERATIONS

1 pair of McIndoe (or other long curved) scissors.
18 Dunhill or Spencer Wells forceps.
6 longer forceps (such as Down Bros.).
6 large Kocher's forceps.
6 Maingot's hysterectomy clamps.
4 Littlewood's (or similar) tissue forceps.
2 needle holders.
1 probe.
1 aneurysm needle.
1 Volkmann's spoon.
2 Vulsellum forceps.
1 uterine holder.
Assorted retractors, including self-retaining ones.
1 Bladder retractor.
3 long sponge-holding forceps.
3 short sponge-holding forceps.
6 towel clips.
2 cross-action clips for securing flexes or the sucker tube.
1 catgut breaker.
Needles, ligatures and suture materials.

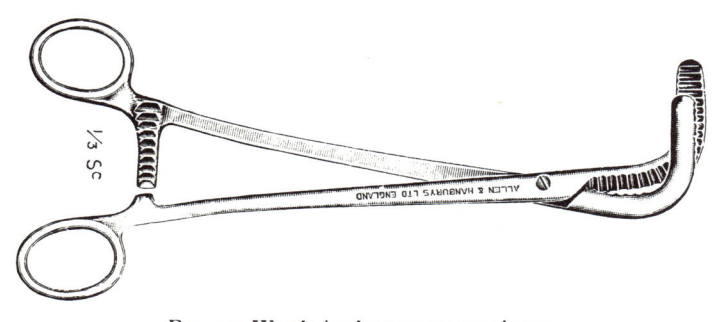

FIG. 77. Wertheim hysterectomy clamp.

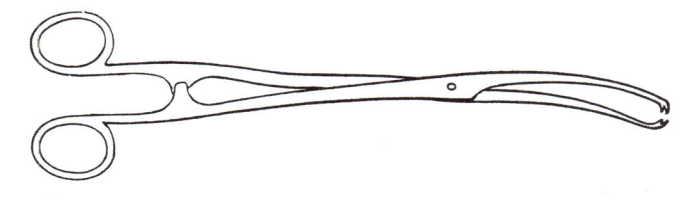

FIG. 78. Vulsellum forceps.

VAGINAL FOUNDATION SET

2 Bard Parker handles and blades.
2 pairs of toothed dissecting forceps.
2 pairs of plain dissecting forceps.
1 pair of long dissecting forceps.
2 pairs of surgeon's straight scissors.
18 pressure forceps.
6 small Kocher's forceps.
6 long pressure forceps.
4 pairs of tissue forceps.
1 silver probe.
1 Volkmann's spoon.
3 small sponge-holding forceps for cleaning skin.
2 needle holders.
1 bladder sound.
1 uterine sound.
1 double-ended curette.
1 bladder retractor.
1 Auvard's speculum.
1 Sims' speculum.
1 set Hegar's dilators.
1 pair of packing forceps.
2 Volsellum forceps.
12 cross action towel clips.
Catgut breaker; needles and suture materials.

FIG. 79. Landon's bladder retractor.

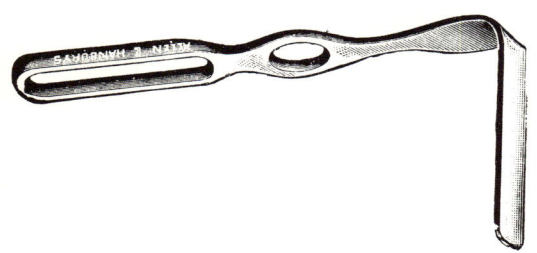

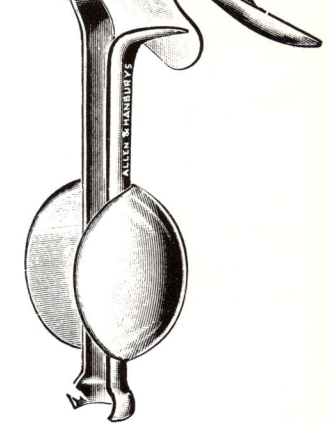

FIG. 80. Auvard's speculum.

DILATION AND CURETTAGE OF THE UTERUS

Instruments

6 towel clips.
2 Volsellum forceps.
1 uterine sound.

GYNÆCOLOGICAL OPERATIONS

1 bladder sound.
1 pair small ovum forceps.
1 double-ended curette.
1 pair of packing forceps.
1 pair of toothed dissecting forceps.
1 pair of long plain dissecting forceps.
1 pair of surgeon's stitch scissors.
1 silver probe.
3 short sponge-holders.
1 Auvard's speculum.
1 Sims' speculum.
1 bladder retractor.
1 set Hegar's dilators.
4 in. gauze roll.
No. 8 plastic catheter and spigot.
Specimen jar.
Pitocin, ergometrine, syntocinon and syringe.

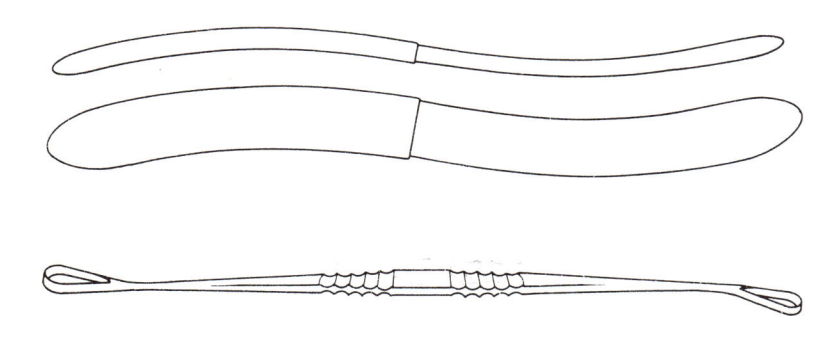

Fig. 81.

This operation entails the gradual dilatation of the cervix until it will admit a curette, with which the interior of the uterus is scraped. It may be performed for these reasons:—

(1) For diagnostic purposes. Suspected carcinoma is the most important condition for which it is used, and in unexplained cases of irregular prolonged or heavy uterine bleeding it should always be performed, even though clinical examination reveals no growth. Curettage may also be used in the investigation of infertility.

(2) For therapeutic reasons. These are less numerous to-day than formerly, but mucous polyps can be removed from the uterine cavity in this way, and the patients with intractable dysmenorrhœa can be treated by dilation of the cervix. In the latter, curettage is not performed unless it is desired to examine the endometrium.

(3) To remove retained products of conception. The uterus in such patients is soft and friable, and a blunt not a sharp curette should be used, lest the uterine wall be perforated. Digital removal is often easier and safer.

The patient is anæsthetized, placed in the lithotomy position and sterile coverings adjusted. A pelvic examination is undertaken while she is anæsthetized. A speculum is introduced, and Sims' may be used if Auvard's is thought too heavy and big for this particular patient. The cervix is pulled down with volsellum forceps, painted with antiseptic, and a uterine sound may be introduced to determine the length and direction of the uterine cavity. The cervix is dilated slowly to avoid tearing until size 8 or 10 of Hegar's dilators has been introduced. A pad of gauze is placed in the vagina to catch the curettings, and with a blunt or sharp curette the whole of the uterine cavity is carefully scraped. It may be possible to gain much information by inspecting the curettings, after which they are transferred to fixative and sent to the pathologist.

Although this is a minor procedure, it opens a pathway for infection to the uterus. The patient may get up for toilet purposes the following day, and may bathe on the second day after operation. A sterile pad is worn until bleeding ceases, and douching must be avoided.

SALPINGECTOMY FOR ECTOPIC GESTATION

Instruments

Abdominal foundation set.
No. 3 soft rubber catheter.
Canney Ryle squirt.
Blood transfusion trolley.

A blood transfusion is begun, the bladder is catheterized, the patient placed in the Trendelenburg position, and a midline incision made. Free blood in the peritoneal cavity is aspirated, and the affected tube identified and drawn out of the wound. It is clamped and removed, blood clot is removed from the Pouch of Douglas, and the abdomen closed. The condition of the patient improves in a remarkable way as soon as the tube is secured and the abdomen closed, but unless her pulse and blood pressure now warrant her return to the ward she should be kept on the table in

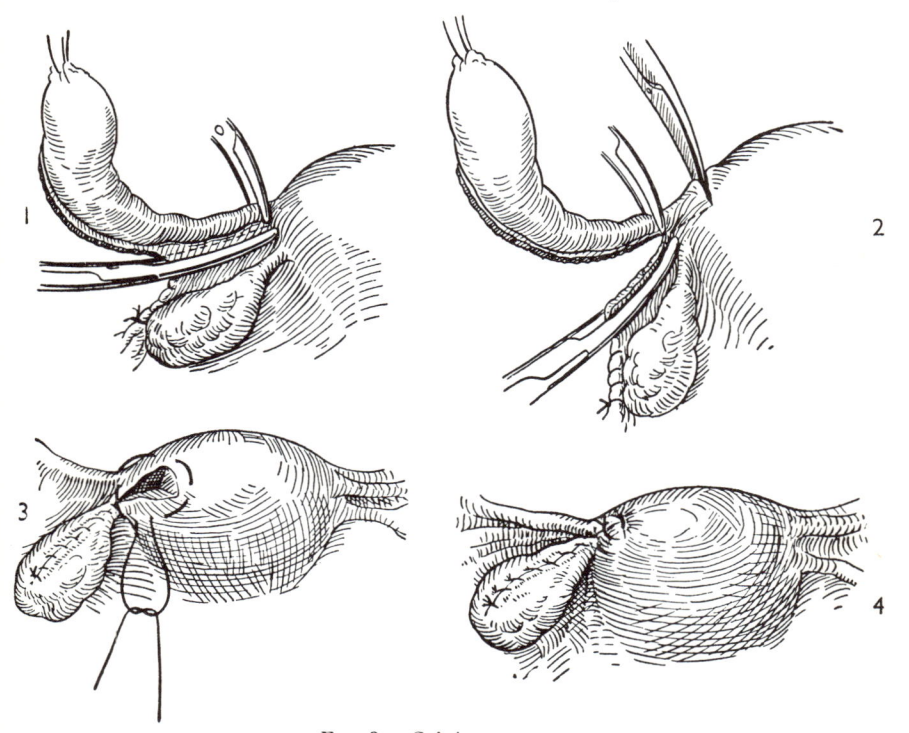

FIG. 82. Salpingectomy.
1. The broad ligament is divided. Notice that the ovary is not removed.
2. The tube is clamped. 3. The cut edges are sutured. 4. Operation completed.

the Trendelenburg position and the blood transfusion continued until she is fit to move.

Salpingectomy or salpingo-oöphorectomy is also performed for chronic salpingitis with pyo- or hydrosalpinx. Such operations take much longer than the one described above since adhesions to adjacent organs may be dense and numerous. The theatre nurse should be prepared to have the gynæcologist perform some operation of his choice for retroversion of the uterus, which is frequently bound down to the Pouch of Douglas. In the presence of uterine disease he might even decide that hysterectomy was needed. The nurse will notice the care taken to cover raw areas in the pelvis, to which loops of intestine might adhere, causing intestinal obstruction.

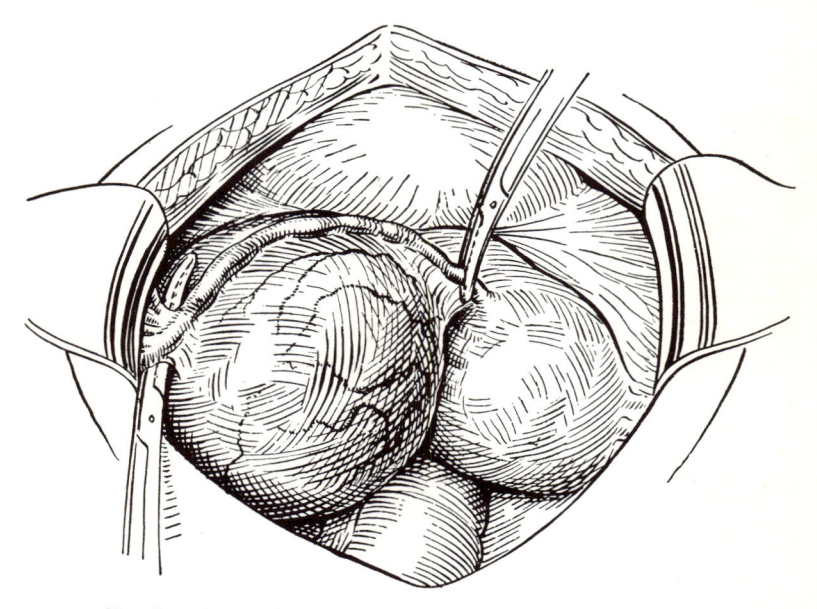

FIG. 83. An ovarian cyst exposed at operation. If any normal ovarian tissue remains, ovarian cystectomy is performed.

OVARIAN CYSTECTOMY

Instruments

Abdominal foundation set.
Ovarian trocar and cannula.

The operation is conducted in the Trendelenburg position, and if the cyst is a big one an incision of generous length is made, since it is undesirable to tap the cyst before removal, in case it proves to be malignant, and the peritoneal cavity is contaminated with its contents. The cyst is first examined, then the opposite ovary and the uterus, and if the growth appears innocent it is drawn out of the wound and the ovarian ligament clamped. If normal ovarian

GYNÆCOLOGICAL OPERATIONS

tissue is present, the cyst is dissected free and removed, or if it has a pedicle this is clamped and divided. An ovarian cyst that has undergone torsion is treated in the same way.

FOTHERGILL'S OPERATION

Instruments

Vaginal foundation set.
3 long Kocher's forceps.
3 Moynihan's forceps.
Infiltration with saline and adrenalin may be needed.

This is a very popular operation in this country for prolapse. When properly performed subsequent pregnancy and delivery following it need not be complicated providing an episiotomy is performed.

The cervix is first dilated, and if it is thought necessary the uterus may also be curetted. The incision passes up the anterior vaginal wall and divides to enclose the cervix, which is amputated. The transverse cervical ligaments are sutured together in front of the uterus, and the raw area is covered by vaginal flaps. Repair of the anterior and posterior vaginal walls and perineum follows. The amputation of the cervix is an advantage if the cervix is lacerated.

Following this operation, patients past the menopause may be worried at the vaginal bleeding that occurs for a day or two, and ask if the periods are returning. They can be told that the bleeding will rapidly cease. The dilation of the cervix is a very important step, since it not only allows curettage, but enables the raw area to be more easily covered with epithelium. If this is not efficiently done, adhesions may seal the orifice and cause retention of secretions. Should these become infected, the uterus may fill with pus to form a PYOMETRA.

VAGINAL HYSTERECTOMY FOR PROLAPSE

Instruments

Vaginal foundation set.
Uterine holder.
6 large Kocher's forceps.
6 large clamps.
3 Moynihan's clamps.

186 MODERN GYNÆCOLOGY FOR NURSES

Vaginal hysterectomy is an operation the popularity of which fluctuates. It is not now often used for the treatment of fibroids, but where uterine disease is accompanied

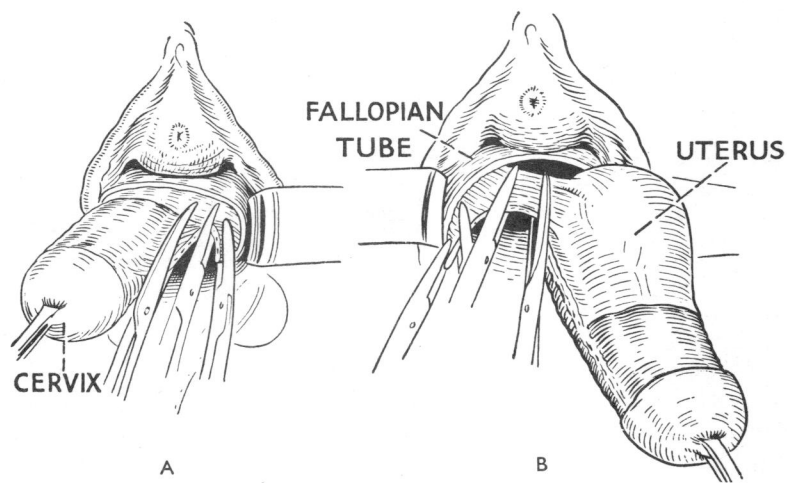

FIG. 84. Vaginal hysterectomy.
(A.) The cervix is drawn down and the vault of the vagina divided.
(B.) The uterus is freed by dividing the transverse and broad ligaments and the Fallopian tubes.

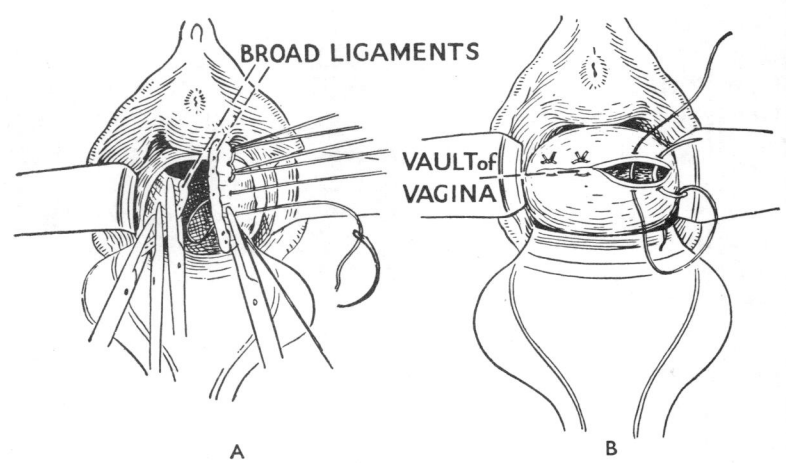

FIG. 85. Vaginal hysterectomy continued.
(A.) The cut tissues from each side of the uterus are sutured together.
(B.) The vault of the vagina is sutured.

by prolapse, the uterus may be removed and the prolapse repaired at the same time, and the operation described by Mayo and Ward is employed. Complete prolapse or procidentia can also be treated by vaginal hysterectomy.

The operation is performed in the lithotomy position. The incision is made into the vault of the vagina and the uterus drawn down and removed. The space occupied by the uterus is closed by drawing together the ovarian and round ligaments and the cut ends of the Fallopian tubes, and the transverse ligaments and utero sacral ligaments. Both the anterior and posterior walls normally need plastic repair with removal of redundant vaginal tissue.

ABDOMINAL TOTAL HYSTERECTOMY

Instruments

Abdominal foundation set.

Removal of the uterus by the abdominal route is most often practised for fibroids. Formerly in many such patients a subtotal hysterectomy would have been performed, the body of the uterus being removed and the cervix left. This operation has fallen into disfavour with gynæcologists to-day, although it is easy to perform, because of the risk of carcinoma developing in the cervical stump.

When the abdomen is open retractors are inserted and the intestines packed away with gauze. The uterus is drawn first to one side and the ovarian ligament and round ligament and tube clamped and divided, then the procedure repeated on the opposite side. The peritoneum over the bladder is opened, the bladder and ureters separated from the upper part of the vagina, and the uterine vessels secured and divided, the greatest care being taken to avoid injury to the ureters. The vagina is first opened posteriorly for this reason with scissors, and the procedure continued till the uterus is freed. A gauze pack may be pushed into the vagina from above to prevent soiling of the peritoneum. Bleeding points are secured, and raw surfaces covered by suture of the peritoneum. The top of the vagina is usually closed, but an opening may be left to allow drainage if there has been much oozing.

The theatre nurse will be impressed in this, and all other types of hysterectomy, with the care with which the surgeon identifies and preserves the ureters.

188 MODERN GYNÆCOLOGY FOR NURSES

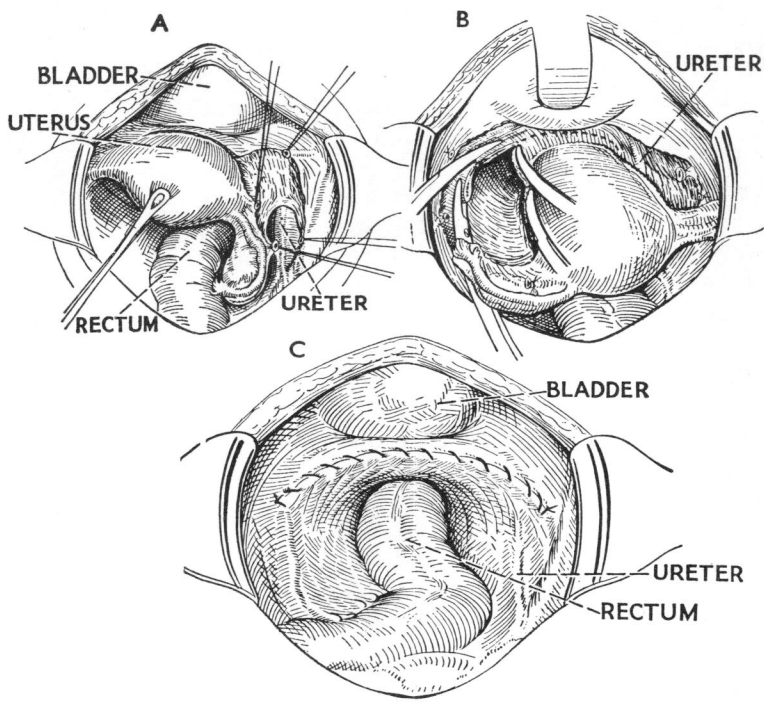

FIG. 86. Total hysterectomy with bilateral salpingo-oöphorectomy.
A. The tissues on either side of the uterus are divided.
B. The bladder is pushed down and the uterus freed by cutting around the vault of the vagina.
C. The operation completed. The raw area has been covered with peritoneum.

WERTHEIM'S HYSTERECTOMY

Instruments

3 Moynihan's clamps.
1 Wertheim clamp.
1 pair Wertheim scissors.
2 Pozze retractors.
3 large sponge-holding forceps.
2 long needle holders.
1 pair of 10 in. toothed dissecting forceps.
1 pair of plain dissecting forceps.
1 long aneurysm needle.
1 pair of McIndoe scissors.
2 small intestinal clamps.

Silver clip magazine and applicators.
Diathermy.

Since this operation is invariably performed for malignant disease, operative difficulties are often greatly increased by the fixation of tissues by the growth. With modern anæsthetic technique, adequate transfusion facilities and better defence against sepsis it has gained in popularity.

The uterus, both tubes and ovaries are removed, together with as much parametrium as possible. This involves stripping the ureters throughout most of their course in the pelvis, and if this is done too thoroughly, sloughing may occur on the tenth day, while if it is not done well, malignant tissue may be left behind. The vagina is dissected clear of the rectum and bladder, and a Wertheim clamp placed as low down over the vagina as possible, to prevent dissemination of cancer cells, and the vagina divided and packed. Glands are removed as widely as possible, and peritoneum is sutured over the raw area. Throughout the operation blood is given.

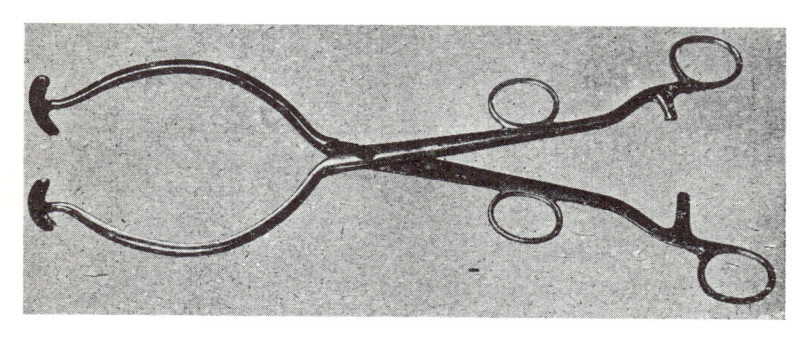

FIG. 87. Berkeley Bonney clamps.

A more extensive operation has been described (Howkins, 1951) in which a synchronous combined abdominoperineal resection is performed, with two surgeons working in the same way as in performing the similar operation on the rectum. The surgeon working from the vagina, with the patient in the lithotomy-Trendelenburg position, makes a circular incision round the vagina and separates it from the urethra and rectum. An indwelling catheter is inserted at the end of the operation, and continuous drainage is used for at least seven days.

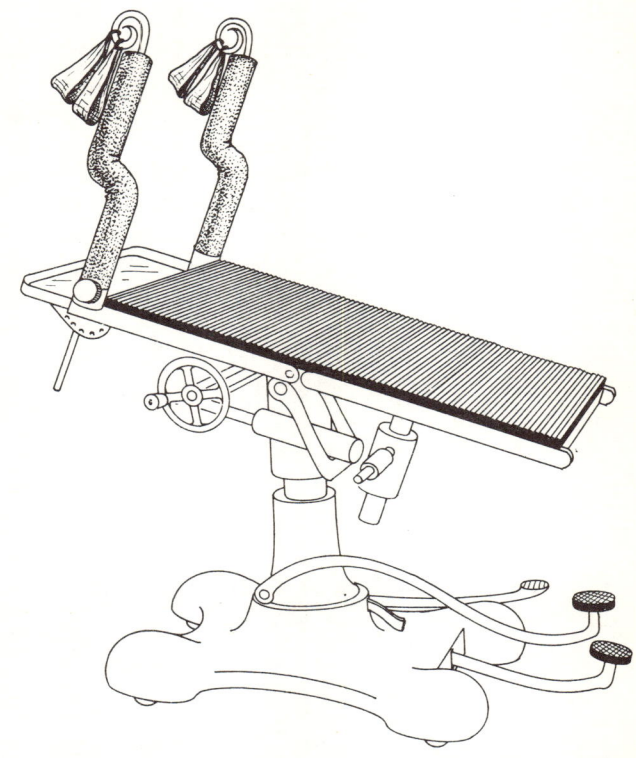

FIG. 88. Theatre table adjusted for an operation in the lithotomy-Trendelenburg position.

PELVIC EXTENTERATION

Still more extensive operations have been devised for the control of widespread malignant growth. If the bladder is involved the ureters may be divided and implanted into the sigmoid colon, and the bladder, uterus and appendages removed. Urine and fæces are then voided per rectum.

If the rectum has been invaded as well, this too has been removed, and the sigmoid colon brought to the surface as a terminal colostomy, to discharge both urine and fæces. This is the so-called " wet " colostomy, and the problems connected with its management are considerable.

The management of a "wet" colostomy presents such a formidable problem to patient and nurse that surgeons have devised an alternative operation when removal of rectum, bladder and reproductive organs is performed in which 6 in. of the terminal ileum is isolated from the small bowel, and into this the ureters are implanted. This isolated segment, or ileal bladder, is sealed by suture at one end, while the other is brought out as a permanent ileostomy through the right side of the abdominal wall. Urine passes down the ureters into this ileal loop, and is collected in a plastic bag.

The advantages of this operation are:

(1) There is no contamination of the loop by bowel contents, so that danger of infection ascending from the ureter to the kidney is reduced. Thus ascending infection is an ever-present risk when the ureters are implanted in the sigmoid colon.

(2) The absorption of electrolytes (e.g. chloride) from the bowel is reduced to a safe level. When the ureters are implanted in the colon all the urine passed by the patient enters the bowel, and a large part of it (water, chlorides and other salts) is reabsorbed into the bloodstream. This reabsorption leads to chemical imbalance and hyperacidity, which is distressing and dangerous to the patient. This condition is called acidosis, and is always a risk in uretero-sigmoid anastomosis, but is averted by the isolated ileal-loop technique.

(3) It can be expected that in most cases careful bowel management will result in a regular daily action of the colostomy in the left flank. Early morning activity and the first meal of the day should initiate the gastro-colic reflex, which causes mass peristalsis in the colon when food enters the stomach and an evacuation of the bowel. Careful regulation of the diet and the fluid intake should be sufficient to ensure a daily action. Foods that are found to cause looseness of the stools or produce flatus should be avoided.

Such operations carry a high mortality, but the limiting factor to their use is not the skill of the surgeon, but the fortitude of the patient in facing life with such a disability, and in England they are not at this time frequently performed.

192 MODERN GYNÆCOLOGY FOR NURSES

The surgeon feels that he aims not merely to preserve life, but that the life must be one that the patient can endure.

CÆSAREAN SECTION

Instruments
Abdominal foundation set.
1 pair of Willett's forceps.
1 pair of Wingley's obstetrical forceps, or those of the surgeon's choice.
2 ml. syringe, and ergometrine and pitocin.
For Baby. Warm sterile towels.
Mucus extractor.

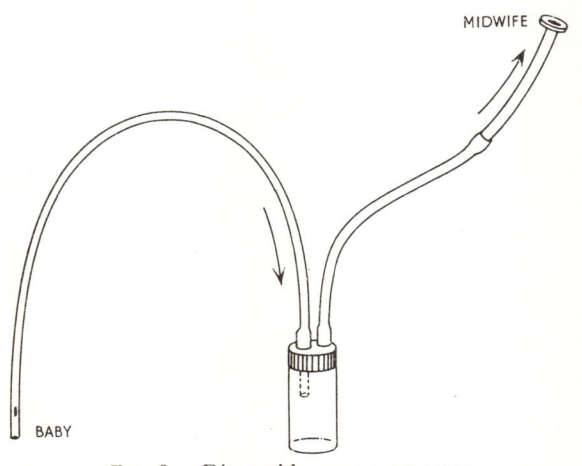

Fig. 89. Disposable mucus extractor.
(*Reproduced from "Obstetrics for Pupil Midwives,"*
S. Bender, Heinemann.)

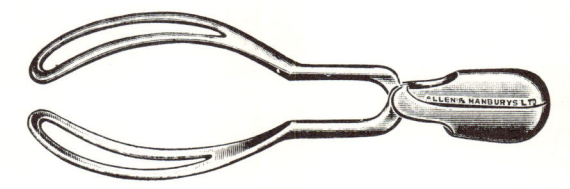

Fig. 90. Wingley's low-cavity obstetrical forceps.

Nasal catheter.
Muslin mouth swabs
Wool eye swabs.
2 ml. syringe.

GYNÆCOLOGICAL OPERATIONS

Lobeline, nalorphine and coramine.
Small face mask to attach to oxygen and carbon dioxide cylinder.
Diluted brandy.

There are two main ways in which the uterus may be opened to deliver a baby by Cæsarean section. The classical incision is a longitudinal one in the upper part of the uterus, by which the baby can be delivered speedily and easily. It has the disadvantage that rupture of the uterus may occur if the patient is allowed to go into normal labour at a subsequent pregnancy. The more usual incision to-day is a transverse one into the lower uterine segment, which is exposed by dividing the peritoneum between the uterus and bladder and retracting the bladder. Extraction of the child is a little more difficult.

The abdomen is opened, and the lower uterine segment exposed as indicated; a hand is introduced and the head delivered, when the rest of the baby follows easily. The cord is clamped and divided, and the child handed to the midwife who in gown and gloves is waiting to receive and resuscitate it. Sometimes it begins to cry at once, but usually a little more time is needed to establish respiration. The use of the head-low position, clearing the air passages with a mucus catheter, or intubation may be indicated.

Meanwhile 0·5 mgm. of ergometrine or an ampoule of syntometrine has been injected intravenously and the uterus contracts and expels the placenta, which is examined by the surgeon, who assures himself that nothing has been left behind. The uterus is sutured with catgut and bleeding controlled. The abdomen is then closed, and an abdominal dressing and perineal pad put on.

This operation is popular with the theatre nurses, who are inclined to miss in theatres the human interest of the wards. It is usually a story with a happy ending as well as a touch of drama, and to send back to the ward a baby alive and crying is a pleasant change from the despatch of unconscious patients from the theatre table.

LAPAROSCOPY

This procedure enables the gynæcologist to inspect the pelvic organs by inserting the laparoscope through the

194 MODERN GYNÆCOLOGY FOR NURSES

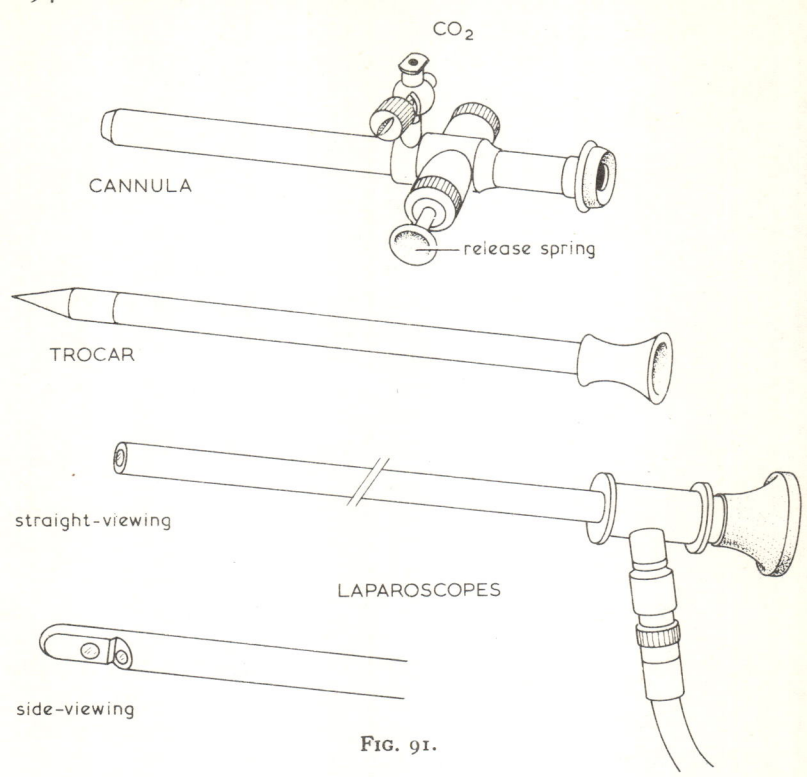

FIG. 91.

abdominal wall, in much the same way as the chest surgeon uses the thoracoscope. Biopsy can be undertaken, and sterilization can be effected by cautery of the Fallopian tubes. Abdominal shave, a Cidal soap bath, and emptying of the bladder and also of the bowel by enema or suppository is required before operation, for which a general anæsthetic is used. Only one skin clip is needed to close the puncture, and this is removed at 24 or 48 hours. Some referred shoulder pain can occur, because of collection under the diaphragm of the nitrous oxide gas which is injected into the peritoneal cavity during laparoscopy. The patient attends the out-patient department later for follow-up and to hear the results of the investigation.

Culdoscopy is a somewhat similar procedure, in which the instrument is passed through the posterior fornix of the vagina with the patient in the knee-elbow position. It is being superseded by laparoscopy.

CHAPTER 12
PREGNANCY

PREGNANCY is a physiological event that occurs without any untoward incident in the lives of many women, and though a textbook must relate at some length the pathological aspects of pregnancy, these are not the ones most frequently met. Most women enjoy excellent health throughout their pregnancies.

The classical first symptom of pregnancy is missing a period, and ten to fourteen days later confirmation may be made by one of the pregnancy tests. These all depend on the fact that the chorionic villi produce, directly or indirectly, large amounts of hormone that is gonadotropic, or gonad-stimulating in action, and that this hormone is excreted in the urine. This hormone appears in the urine in significant amounts a week after the first missed period. The level rises to its peak in ten weeks, declines to the twentieth week, and does not entirely disappear until after delivery.

PREGNANCY TESTS

Biological tests, involving the use of laboratory animals, have now been entirely replaced by immunological techniques. The urine specimen used is preferably an early morning one, since this is the most concentrated, and therefore contains the largest amount of human chorionic gonadotrophin (HCG). The receptacle used should be free from any trace of detergent, which may falsify the result. Infected or very cloudy urine is not suitable for testing, and some methods cannot be used if protein is present.

The commonest test requires two reagents, an HCG antiserum, and either latex particles or red blood cells coated with HCG. If urine from a non-pregnant woman is added to the HCG antiserum, this is not neutralized and remains active; if some of the HCG-coated particles are added to it, flocculation occurs. Should the urine contain HCG, however, this will neutralize the HCG antibodies, and when the HCG coated particles are added, no reaction takes place, and this is the positive or pregnancy-confirming result. The percentage of errors in the result is very low if the test is carefully performed, and if it is not undertaken too early in pregnancy, or following an abortion.

These tests are only used if the earliest diagnosis of pregnancy must be made or excluded. There are of course many social as well as personal reasons why this information may be important early, and advertisement of pregnancy testing services to the general public indicates the demand that exists for this knowledge.

All pregnancy tests become positive about ten days after the first missed period, and remain positive for about forty-eight hours after delivery. The rare conditions **vesicular mole and chorion epithelioma** (p. 236), **also** produce a positive result, the hormone being present in amounts 200 times greater than normal, so that even if the urine is diluted to the diagnostic level of 1 in 200, a positive result will still be obtained.

ANATOMY

The basic problem of midwifery is that the baby at term must be pushed by the contracting uterus through the bony ring of the pelvis and the soft parts that form the pelvic floor. The structure of the pelvis must be studied because the shape, size and direction of the birth canal determine the way in which the baby is born.

The pelvis is formed by three bones: the two innominate bones meet anteriorly at the symphysis pubis and are separated posteriorly by the sacrum. The latter is **triangular**, formed by five fused vertebræ that diminish in size towards the junction with the coccyx below. The upper border, the sacral promontory, is a very important landmark in the pelvis, and a broad sacrum makes the pelvis roomy.

The innominate bone is formed from three parts which unite at the acetabulum, or socket, that forms part of the hip-joint. The three parts are:—

(*a*) The ilium is the wide upper part. The nurse who gives intramuscular injections into the buttocks has learned to identify its upper margin, the iliac crest, which ends anteriorly in the anterior iliac spine. Posteriorly the ileum

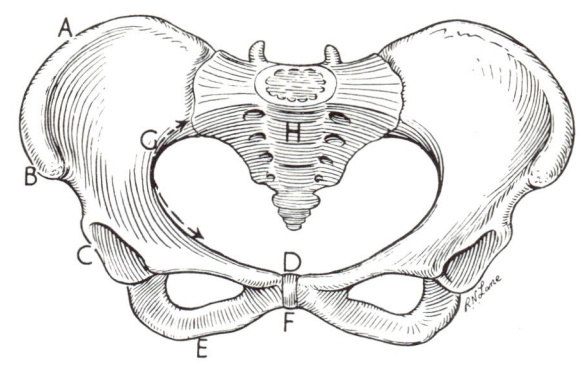

FIG. 92. The female pelvis.
A. Iliac crest.
B. Anterior superior iliac spine.
C. Acetabulum.
D. Symphisis pubis.
E. Ischial tuberosity.
F. Sub-pubic arch.
G. Ilio-pectineal line (pelvic brim).
H. Sacrum.

forms a joint with the sacrum, and inferiorly it forms the sciatic notch through which the sciatic nerve leaves the pelvis for the leg.

(b) The ischium is the lowest part of the innominate bone and its most important feature is the ischial tuberosity, a thick bony process on which one sits and which forms one of the boundaries of the pelvic outlet.

(c) The pubis is the anterior portion which meets its fellow in front at the symphysis pubis. This is a cartilaginous joint which softens during pregnancy enabling the bones to separate slightly and, therefore, increase the diameter of the pelvis a little. The angle made by two bones at the inferior margin of the symphysis pubis and known as the sub-pubic arch is normally more than a right angle. This allows the baby's head to come well forward beneath the symphysis during birth and avoid damage to the perineum.

If the bony pelvis is inspected from above, it will be seen that, from the sacral promontory, a well-marked ridge runs forward on each side towards the symphysis pubis. This is the ilio-pectineal line and the circle thus formed constitutes the brim or inlet of the true pelvis. The pelvic inlet forms the beginning of the birth canal and its size and shape influence the course of labour profoundly.

If the pelvis is looked at from below, the bony boundaries of the outlet are seen to be the coccyx, the pubic angle and the ischial tuberosities. The outlet which is slightly larger than the inlet is unlikely to cause any difficulty if the baby has passed through the pelvic brim without incident.

The pelvic outlet is closed by the two levator ani muscles which slope downwards and forwards. There are two openings in the muscular floor of the pelvis, one for the rectum and the other for the vagina and urethra.

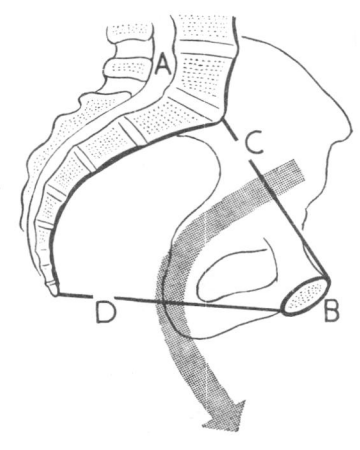

FIG. 93. Section of the female pelvis, showing the curve of the birth canal.
A. Sacrum.
B. Symphysis pubis.
C. Pelvic brim.
D. Pelvic outlet.

If the pelvis is seen in section, it will be noticed that the birth canal has a long posterior wall, formed by the curve of the sacrum, and a short anterior wall, formed by the symphysis pubis. As the baby is born, it is directed forward under the pubic arch both by the slope of the pelvic floor and the forward curvature of the birth canal.

PHYSIOLOGY OF PREGNANCY

Pregnancy begins with the fertilization of the ovum in the outer part of the Fallopian tube (p. 81). Cell division begins almost at once as the fertilized egg-cell passes onwards to the uterus. It divides first into two cells, then into four, and so rapidly becomes a mass of cells said to resemble a mulberry or morula. Differentiation then takes place, the outer layer developing into the nutritional layer or trophoblast, while within this the embryo begins to form. The trophoblast, by the time the ovum reaches the uterus, on the seventh day of its existence, or the twenty-first day of the menstrual cycle, has developed into a layer of minute branching processes, the chorionic villi, which secrete a fluid that can erode the tissues with which they come in contact. The endometrium has thickened into a highly vascular secretory state under the influence of progesterone, and when the ovum enters the uterus it digests for itself a nest in the endometrium into which it embeds itself.

The embedding should take place in the fundus of the uterus; but if it occurs low down in the uterine cavity, trouble will occur during labour from interference with the baby's blood supply before it can be delivered. This abnormal implantation causes the dangerous condition known as placenta prævia. Fortunately this is not common,

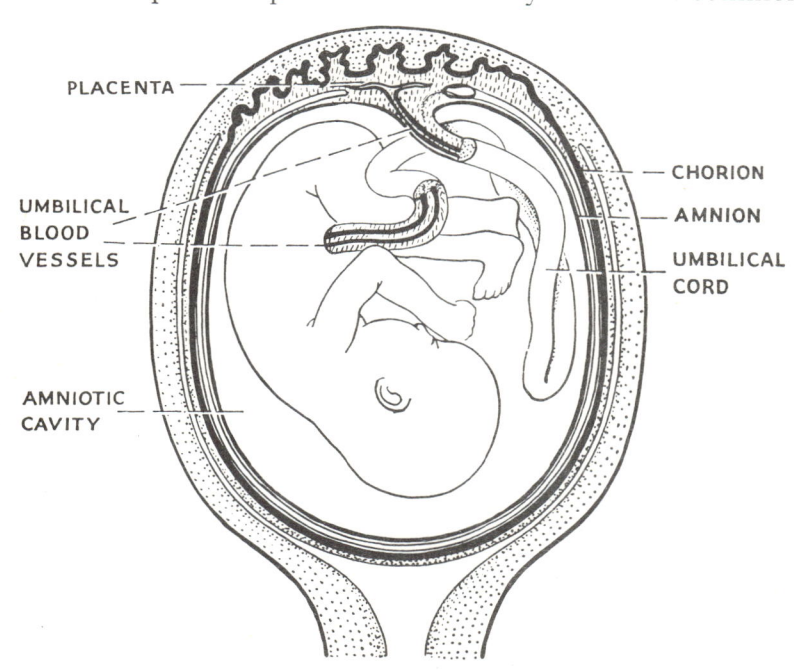

FIG. 94. Developing fetus in utero, showing the placenta and fetal membranes (amnion and chorion).

200 MODERN GYNÆCOLOGY FOR NURSES

since the ovum generally is ready for embedding when it reaches the fundus, and normally neither attaches itself prematurely to the Fallopian tube nor migrates downwards towards the internal os.

Meanwhile the chorionic villi secrete chorionic gonadotrophin. This hormone is not only responsible for the

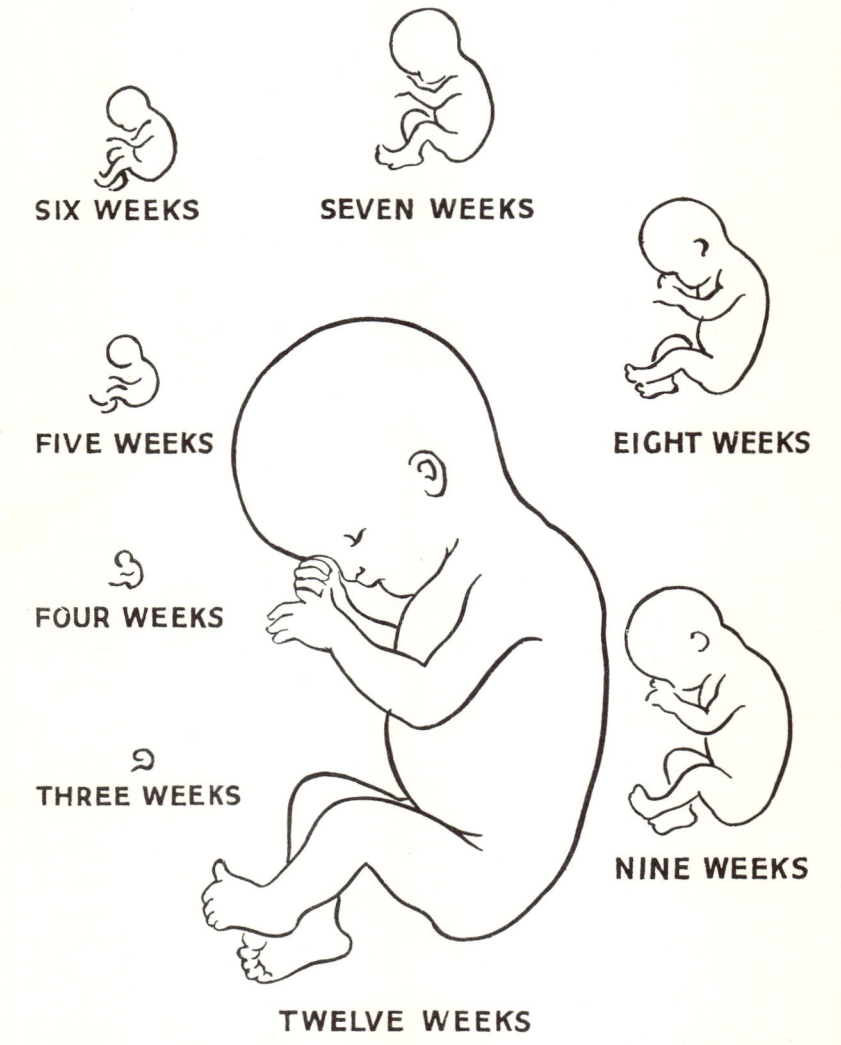

FIG. 95. Size of growing fetus at successive stages of pregnancy.
(from "Childbirth Without Fear," G. Dick-Read, Heinemann.)

positive pregnancy test, but also stimulates the pituitary to produce more luteinizing hormone (LH), which increases the size and prolongs the life of the corpus luteum in the ovary. The corpus luteum produces increasing amounts of progesterone, so that the period is suppressed, and the endometrium increases rapidly in thickness and vascularity, to be converted into the DECIDUA of pregnancy. The corpus luteum remains active for about three months, when its functions are gradually taken over by the chorionic villi.

The placenta at term is a thick circular disc, 15 to 20 cm. (6 to 8 in.) in diameter, and about 3·5 cm. (1½ in.) thick. This depth is greatest at the centre and least at the periphery. The surface which lies against the uterus is rough, and divided by fissures into about fifteen divisions or cotyledons. The fetal surface is covered by the smooth amnion, and crossed by the blood vessels which converge towards the centre to form the umbilical cord which conveys blood to and from the fetus. There are two umbilical arteries carrying deoxygenated blood from the baby to the placenta, and one umbilical vein taking oxygenated blood from the placenta to the fœtus. These are supported by a semi-solid material, Wharton's jelly, and enclosed in amnion to form a twisted structure up to 60 cm. (2 ft.) long. This is long enough to allow the fetus a range of movement, entering its umbilicus at one end and at the other attached more or less centrally to the placenta.

The functions of the placenta are as follows:—

(1) Oxygen and foodstuffs are supplied to the fetus via the umbilical vein, and waste products, including carbon dioxide, removed via the two umbilical arteries.

(2) As mentioned above, it is an endocrine organ. Chorionic gonadotropin is produced, and also œstrogen and progesterone.

(3) Most viruses and organisms are unable to penetrate the placental barrier. Two important exceptions are syphilis (p. 161) and German measles (rubella) which if contracted by the mother in the first twelve weeks of pregnancy is able to damage the eye and ear of the baby, and cause congenital cataract and deafness.

Some of the mother's antibodies also cross the placenta, so that a baby has a passive immunity to some diseases like measles and mumps for the first few months of its life if the mother is immune to them.

At term contractions of the uterus result in drawing up and dilatation of the cervix. The gestation sac ruptures, and the baby passes down the vagina and is born. Further contractions peel the placenta from the uterus, and this too is expelled with the fetal membranes in which the baby was enclosed adhering to its margins.

FETAL CIRCULATION

The main essentials of fetal development are complete by the twelfth week. Any harmful influences, such as viruses or certain drugs, that reach the fetus from the mother's blood during these early months may cause congenital deformities.

The blood circulation of the fetus is important because a profound change must take place at birth, and anomalies in development may give rise to trouble in post-natal life. Since the baby does not breathe in utero, it does not require a big pulmonary circulation, but it does need a large placental blood-flow, and the fœtal circulation is adapted especially to meet these needs.

Oxygenated blood reaches the fetus from the placenta along the umbilical vein. Most of this blood passes the liver, and reaches the inferior vena cava by means of the ductus venosus. This blood enters the right atrium, and instead of going into the right ventricle and the pulmonary artery, most of it is immediately directed into the left atrium by the foramen ovale. This is a valvular opening in the atrial septum which enables oxygenated blood to be shunted directly into the left side of the heart. In addition, a part of the blood that does enter the pulmonary artery is also diverted into the aorta by the ductus arteriosus.

The brain and the head are supplied by the vessels from the arch of the aorta which contains well-oxygenated blood; the legs from the aorta below the ductus arteriosus, which contains comparatively deoxygenated blood, but they do not in utero require a high concentration of oxygen. Deoxygenated blood returns to the placenta by the two umbilical arteries within the umbilical cord. The lungs expand when the baby takes its first breath, and much larger quantities of blood are needed in the pulmonary arteries.

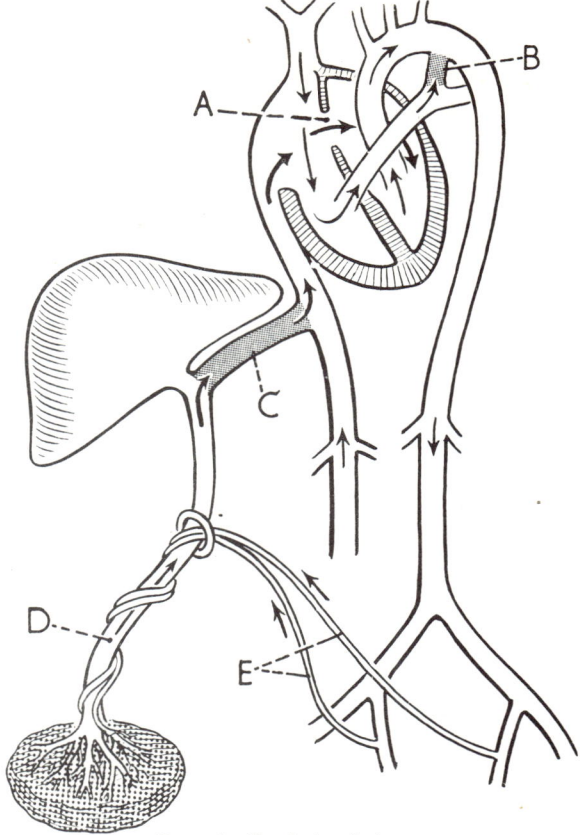

FIG. 96. Fetal circulation.

A. Foramen ovale.
B. Ductus arteriosus.
C. Ductus venosus.
D. Umbilical vein, carrying oxygenated blood from placenta to fœtus.
E. Umbilical arteries, carrying deoxygenated blood back to placenta.

The foramen ovale closes almost immediately, and the ductus arteriosus and ductous venosus close soon after birth. When the cord is tied, clotting occurs in the umbilical vessels and the lungs take over from the placenta the oxygenizing functions that they are to maintain throughout life.

SIGNS AND SYMPTOMS OF PREGNANCY

Pregnancy lasts about 280 days, though periods much in excess of this have been reported, and accepted in the courts. The sequence of events is broadly as follows:—

Amenorrhœa is normal throughout pregnancy, though some women menstruate during the early months of pregnancy without pathological causes. Such losses are usually less than those of a normal period.

Soon after the first missed period, the breasts begin to enlarge, and the patient is conscious of a feeling of congestion. The primary areola becomes more pigmented, especially in dark-haired women, and a secondary areola appears around it. Within the primary areola appear a number of tubercles, from twelve to twenty, and though not diagnostic of pregnancy these Montgomery's tubercles are supporting evidence.

At the eighth week, the cervix will be found to be softer than usual, and the vagina has a violet tint, both changes being due to increasing vascularity.

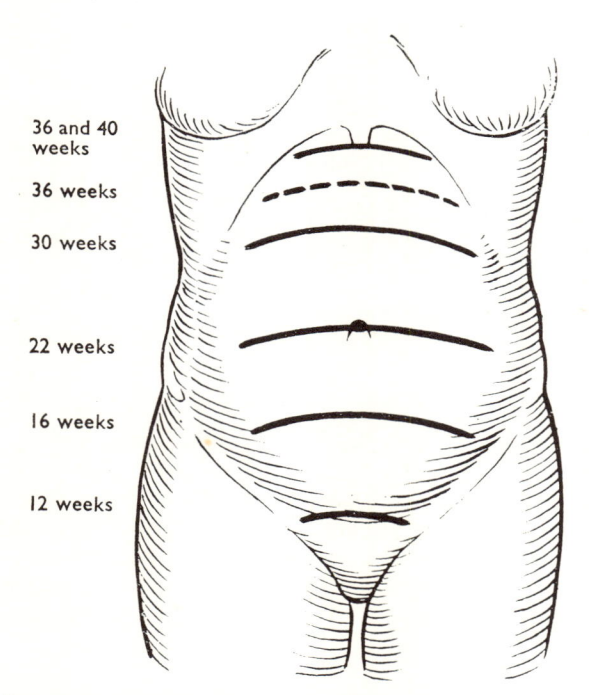

FIG. 97. The height of the fundus at successive stages of pregnancy. It sinks at thirty-six weeks in primigravidæ, when the head engages in the pelvis. In all patients at forty weeks, the fundus reaches approximately to the xiphisternum.

During these weeks some nausea or actual vomiting is common, especially in the mornings. Frequency of micturition is common until the uterus rises out of the pelvis at the fourteenth week.

At the twelfth week the fundus of the uterus can just be felt from the abdomen. A little clear fluid can now be expressed from the breasts, though in some cases this sign occurs earlier. Opalescent fluid in a woman who has had children before is of no significance.

At sixteen weeks the uterus is half way to the umbilicus. If the patient is a multipara, she may recognize the movements of the fetus (commonly known as " quickening "); if it is her first baby, she is usually a little slower in doing so. An X-ray will reveal the fetal bones.

At the twenty-fourth week, the fœtal heart can be heard, and the uterus reaches just above the umbilicus.

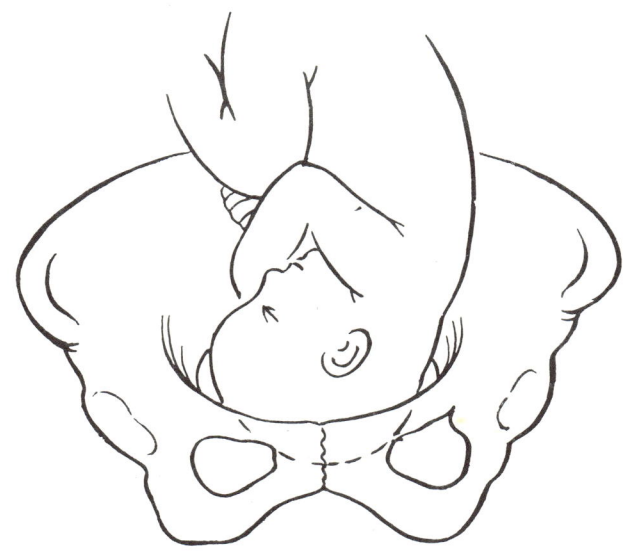

FIG. 98. Engagement of the head. In a primigravida the head usually descends into the pelvis before labour begins.

At thirty-six weeks in a primigravida the presenting part usually engages in the pelvis, and the level of the fundus drops an inch or two. This is the sign of " lightening," and it increases the comfort of the patient very considerably.

ANTENATAL CARE

Statistics tell us that a woman who receives continuous care throughout pregnancy has a far better chance of a safe delivery and a healthy baby than one who does not. She will have peace of mind; she will be able to take such decisions as where to have the baby with due consideration; minor troubles can be treated before they can give rise to major complications; she will be made aware of the benefits and services available to her. She will in addition be receptive at this important time to education in many aspects of physical and mental health, which will be to the benefit of both her baby and herself. Midwives and clinic nurses try to ensure that the patient is well informed, so that pregnancy is serene and a safe delivery is confidently expected.

A patient who believes herself pregnant goes to her doctor for confirmation, and a decision must then be taken as to where she will go for ante-natal care, and eventually for delivery. If this is her first baby, or if there is any medical reason for expecting difficulty, delivery will be in hospital, or in a general practitioner unit with hospital facilities available. Only if she is an entirely healthy woman expecting her second or third baby, and with satisfactory domestic circumstances may her delivery at home be considered. Home confinements are becoming progressively less common. Antenatal care may be supplied by the doctor, if he undertakes obstetric practice, and the clinic nurses, or may be given entirely in the hospital.

Her first visit will be about the eighth week. She is examined, and the expected date of delivery estimated. The quickest method is to count back three months from the beginning of her last period, and add seven days. Thus if her last period began on June 1st, her expected date of delivery will be March 8th, and a bed will be booked for her.

At this attendance a history is taken, and its importance cannot be overstressed. A history of rheumatic fever will suggest the possibility of mitral valve disease, of which the commonest form is stenosis. A heart with such a handicap may enable the patient to support normal activities without symptoms, but the additional strain of pregnancy may precipitate heart failure. Maternal mortality in such cases is not inconsiderable, and most careful medical and nursing supervision will be necessary. Other examples of important items in the medical history are scarlet fever, pulmonary tuberculosis and diabetes, all of which may cause complications during pregnancy or labour.

If there has been a previous confinement an accurate history of any abnormal event may be rewarding. A story of toxæmia of pregnancy is important because there is an increased risk in succeeding pregnancies of its recurrence. A long labour ending in a forceps delivery may suggest a small maternal pelvis; a history of a difficult delivery ending in a stillbirth is even more suggestive of disproportion between the baby and the mother's pelvis, and this is doubly significant if the weight of the baby was 7 lb. or less.

A complete physical examination is performed with special attention directed to the condition of the teeth and gums and the colour of the mucus membranes. The heart and lungs are carefully examined to exclude any previously unknown disease. The breasts and nipples are inspected so that advice may be given regarding breast feeding. The abdomen is examined especially to assess the size of the uterus and pelvic examination is performed to confirm the presence and normality of the pregnancy, as well as to exclude abnormalities such as ovarian cysts. The size and contents of the bony pelvis are noted and the vagina and cervix inspected with a speculum for the presence of vaginal discharge or cervical erosion. The legs are inspected for œdema or the presence of varicose veins.

INVESTIGATION. The *chest* is X-rayed only if there is a special indication because radiography is used, radiography is used with caution during pregnancy lest the fetus suffer, and the pelvis is not X-rayed without good grounds for doing so. The *urine* is examined (especially for albumin, acetone and sugar), and the *blood pressure* and *weight* recorded at this and every visit. Blood examinations include the *hæmoglobin level*, *blood group* and *Rhesus* type, while the *Wassermann* or some similar test is undertaken to detect untreated syphilis that might affect the baby. She is referred to the *dentist*, since the increasing needs of the fetus for calcium may cause a deterioration in the mother's teeth.

The Rhesus factor referred to above is present in the blood of 85% of the population in the British Isles, and these are spoken of as Rhesus positive (Rh +) while the minority are said to be Rhesus negative (Rh —). This factor is inherited by the children as a Mendelian dominant. If both parents are Rh — or both are Rh + so are all the children. A Rh — woman married to a Rh + man who is homozygous for this factor will have children all of whom are Rh +.

Unfortunately the Rhesus factor is an antigen, and if Rh + cells gain access to the circulation of a Rh — person, she will make antibodies to Rh + cells, and the presence of this antibody in the blood can be detected by means of Coombs' test. There are two ways in which this sensitization can take place. (1) By an incompatible blood transfusion, which should now be a very rare occurrence. (2) By the conception by a Rh — woman of a Rh + fetus. The amount of antibody in her blood will increase with successive pregnancies, until it is sufficient to cause breakdown, or hæmolysis, of the cells of the Rh + fœtus *in utero*. A severely affected child may be born dead; in a less severe case the baby suffers soon after birth from anæmia and hæmolytic jaundice, which may be fatal unless adequately treated.

If a pregnant woman is Rh —, and her husband is Rh +, she will probably give birth to a Rh + infant which will sensitize her so that she will develop Rh antibodies during her second and subsequent pregnancies. These antibodies will increase in amount with each pregnancy and as each pregnancy progresses so that frequent estimation of the Rh antibody level in the blood are essential during pregnancy. These levels give an indication of the condition of the affected fetus.

A more accurate method for estimating the condition of the fetus is amniocentesis, which is discussed at the end of this section. Very mildly affected babies will be delivered at or just before term whilst the severely affected ones will be delivered at thirty-five or thirty-six weeks. In all cases preparation is made to give the baby immediately after birth an exchange blood transfusion, removing from the baby its own corpuscles and substituting an equal volume of Rh — blood. Such a transfusion will enable the baby to survive until the antibody in its bloodstream is eliminated. A second or third transfusion may be necessary if a high serum bilirubin level indicates that hæmolysis is still taking place.

Intrauterine Transfusion. Some babies are unfortunately so severely affected that they die *in utero* before the thirty-fifth week of pregnancy. Amniocentesis will determine when this tragedy is about to happen and in some instances it can be prevented by giving the baby a transfusion of Rh — cells whilst it remains in the uterus and the pregnancy continues. The technique is highly specialized and performed in only a few obstetric units. Under very careful X-ray control the position of the baby is accurately defined and a long needle is introduced through the mother's anterior abdominal wall, through the uterus until it passes through the abdominal wall of the baby to enter the peritoneal cavity. Rhesus — red cells are then injected into the baby's peritoneal cavity and the needle is withdrawn. The red cells are absorbed into the circulation of the fetus and keep it alive. This procedure may have to be repeated several times before delivery at the thirty-fifth week.

Anti-D Globulin. It is now possible to prevent a woman being sensitized by her Rh + infant. Sensitization takes place immediately after delivery when Rh + cells from the fetus enter the mother's circulation where they can be detected by a special test. Blood is therefore taken from all Rh — women about thirty minutes after delivery to be tested for circulating Rh + cells from the fetus. If any are present the mother is given Anti-D Globulin which will immediately destroy them and so prevent the mother developing antibodies and having an affected baby in her next pregnancy.

Rh — patients feel justifiable anxiety about the effect of their blood group on their unborn infant, but the nurse can assure them that the outlook is not as bad as the lay public believes. The first pregnancy is not affected and neither are later ones if effective treatment is given: the husband may be heterozygous for the factor so that some children may be Rh — and unaffected; and exchange transfusion is an effective treatment if a baby is born with hæmolytic anæmia.

ADVICE

Diet. In western countries, about two thirds of the daily calorie intake is supplied by carbohydrates such as bread, potatoes, cereals and sweet foods, and one third each by fats and by proteins. The growing fetus draws its requirements from its mother's bloodstream, and needs especially amino acids to make its own proteins; calcium and phosphorus for bones, and iron for red blood cells. Protein foods are the most expensive item in the shopping basket, and women with less to spend than others on housekeeping are likely to go short of these, and to use starchy foods instead, which tend to cause an undesirable weight gain. Realistic advice on what represents the best bargain at the time must be given. Proteins often have a double advantage in the diet; for instance, red meat contains iron and some of the B-vitamins; fish is a source of iodine, necessary for the development of the thyroid gland; while milk and cheese contain calcium. Salads, green vegetables and fruit supply vitamin C, and also the roughage that will help to make constipation less of a problem. Plenty of fluid to drink is important, but sweet drinks which give calories but no extra nutrition should be avoided. If a good mixed diet is being taken, the vitamin requirements are normally being met, but women on a low income may need supplements, and capsules of vitamins A and D may be thought necessary for many during the winter. Fried and heavy foods are to be avoided in the early days because nausea may be a problem, and later in pregnancy when the enlarging uterus may embarrass the stomach and give rise to indigestion.

Strange longings for food sometimes appear in the early months of pregnancy, often for highly flavoured foods, and unless there is something undesirable about the article craved, there is no need to prohibit it, though highly salted foods and excessive weight gain should be discouraged.

Weight Control. The average weight increase should not exceed $\frac{1}{2}$ lb. a week, and any sudden increase in the middle or late weeks suggests a retention of water, which is one of the first signs of toxæmia (p. 218). Apart from this grave complication, the burden of unnecessary weight makes a patient uncomfortable and short of breath, and on the whole a fat woman has a more tedious and difficult labour than a thin one, since she is more readily exhausted by the physical effort. It is also demoralizing for a woman to lose her trimness as a result of having a baby. Unreasonable weight increase is curbed by restriction of salt and carbohydrate consumption, and reliance on moderate intake of first-class protein, fresh fruit and vegetables. Total weight gain throughout pregnancy should not exceed 20 lbs., and an absolute permitted maximum of 28 lbs.

Clothes. Advice on clothes is needed less nowadays, but the patient should be warned against any constriction of the legs by tight stocking-tops which might predispose to varicose veins. Shoes should have low heels, or the effort of balancing on high ones may cause backache or falls. Walking exercises by the physiotherapist may improve the posture in the later months. The brassiere should be a good supporting one that does not compress the nipples. Heavy or stiff corsets are undesirable.

Nipples. A slight secretion from the nipple is normal and this serous fluid tends to dry on the nipple to form scaly crusts. Removal with soap and water is all that is required; vigorous scrubbing damages the skin, and may well lead to complications when lactation starts. It is permissible to lubricate the nipple sparingly with olive oil towards the end of pregnancy, but it is wrong to harden it with surgical spirit.

Activity. Pregnancy is not to be regarded as a period of invalidism, and the expectant mother need curtail her usual routine but little. She should if possible take a reasonably brisk walk daily in the fresh air, and rest in the afternoon for an hour or two with her feet up. She should go to bed early, and avoid excessive social engagements that involve late hours.

Smoking. Women who smoke during pregnancy have babies smaller than the average, and this lower birth weight is associated with higher mortality. It is thought that nicotine constricts the blood vessels, so reducing the supply of oxygenated blood to the baby. Some investigators claim that the harmful effects can be traced even into childhood. There is no safe level of cigarette smoking, and pregnant women should be told very plainly of the risks it carries for the baby, as well as for the mother herself in later life from bronchitis and lung cancer.

Parentcraft classes. Group teaching for mothers-to-be has been expanded to include prospective fathers, who sometimes find that the arrival of the first baby creates unlooked-for problems, unless their role in pregnancy, labour and the puerperium is made clear. Such classes are conducted on an informal basis, with plenty of opportunity to ask questions and explore problems.

REASSURANCE

Available Resources. The National Health Service provides the expectant mother with benefits of which she may not be aware in her first pregnancy. She may have a pint of milk daily at a reduced price, and orange juice, cod-liver oil vitamin and iron tablets can be obtained free or at a nominal charge. Dental treatment is also free.

In addition financial grants are available. The Maternity Grant is a lump sum which can be claimed between three months before delivery and three months afterwards. The Maternity Allowance is paid weekly for eighteen weeks to those women who normally go out to work and who have the necessary stamps on their cards. It enables working women to rest before and after the birth of the baby without undue financial hardship.

A medical social worker will be present in the department, and the patient should be referred to her if help is indicated. Patients may be unmarried, or the husband may be away serving in the forces, or disabled. Perhaps the patient is living in rooms and fears the landlady will not be willing to accept a baby. Many women have a big burden to carry as well as pregnancy and any help that can be given is acceptable.

Subsequently the patient should visit the department once a month. She is weighed, her urine is tested and her blood pressure recorded each time. As pregnancy advances, the position of the fetus in the uterus becomes of increasing importance. The most favourable presentation is by the vertex; that is, the baby's head enters the pelvis first. Should the head be uppermost, it is usual to try to turn the baby round, since breech delivery is more difficult, and carries an increased risk to the baby. If it is impossible to turn it, delivery in hospital rather than at home would be essential.

Classes are held in most antenatal centres to teach exercises that will help strengthen the muscles of the abdomen and pelvic floor. Relaxation as well as contraction of muscles is taught, so that during the early stages of labour when no active efforts by the patient are required, she may rest and prepare for the muscular contractions that are required of her later. Even to-day some women have vague ideas as to the course of labour, and their anxieties can be allayed by careful preparation beforehand.

In hospital it frequently happens that the out-patient department and the labour ward are staffed separately. This has the disadvantage that the patient who knows and trusts the people who looked after her during pregnancy finds that she has an unknown set of attendants when she comes into labour. Where possible, the ward midwives should attend antenatal sessions, and have some contact with their patients before delivery.

At some hospitals the patient visits the labour ward before delivery, and has an opportunity to ask questions. She may have the apparatus used for the relief of pain explained to her, and if she can try the effect of gas and oxygen, she has confidence in its effect later.

With efficient antenatal care, it is hoped that the pregnancy will be uneventful, and that the patient at term is fit and confident of a healthy baby. However, there are some discomforts and troubles that may need treatment, and some major complications to be averted.

AMNIOCENTESIS is an important modern method of fetal monitoring. A specimen of amniotic fluid is withdrawn through an abdominal puncture, and can be used to give a range of information. It is performed under a local anaesthetic, and the size of needle used depends on the amount of fat in the abdominal wall. Amniocentesis may be undertaken early in pregnancy to see if congenital chromosome abnormalities are present, or to determine the sex of a baby. The cases for which this is necessary are few but important, since if a congenital abnormality (such as Down's syndrome) is present, pregnancy can be terminated. Later in pregnancy, examination of skin cells (fetal squames) may be done to determine maturity, or if the baby is likely to suffer from the respiratory distress syndrome if labour has to be induced. If the liquor is to be examined for bilirubin (as in Rhesus iso-immunity), the specimen must be put at once into a dark wrapper, since bilirubin is destroyed by ultraviolet light.

Amnioscopy is the examination of the liquor from outside the membranes by a lighted scope passed through the cervix. The information obtained is slight compared with that gained from amniocentesis.

MINOR COMPLICATIONS

MORNING SICKNESS

Morning sickness is not uncommon during the first three months of pregnancy. The patient feels nausea on awaking, and vomits a little clear mucus. Nausea at other times of day is often experienced, and sometimes vomiting is so severe as to make this a major problem.

The patient should lie still for half an hour after waking in the morning, and if possible should have a cup of tea and a biscuit before rising. The fluid intake should be high, glucose is helpful, and an alkaline mixture can be tried, though quite unscientific. Avomine is often successful in checking vomiting, though more powerful antihistamine drugs may be needed to control severe vomiting. If it is severe, the urine should always be tested for ketones and if any are present the patient should be admitted to hospital.

VARICOSE VEINS

Dilated veins may appear in the legs of a patient who has not previously suffered from them, while those who already possess them find them aggravated. Pressure in the pelvis by the growing fetus is not responsible, since the varicose veins often appear before such pressure can be blamed. Progesterone, which is present in high concentration in the blood, relaxes smooth muscle throughout the body, including that of the veins. The constipation which is common in the early months of pregnancy is due to the same cause.

Active treatment is not indicated. The patient may sleep with the end of the bed raised a few inches, and should rest with the feet up for an hour or so in the middle of the afternoon. Crepe bandages tend to form ridges, and elastic stockings give better support. The newest elastic nylon ones are acceptable even to the most fastidious patient. If the condition does not disappear after delivery, injection or ligature and stripping of the veins may be undertaken.

PREGNANCY

HÆMORRHOIDS

Hæmorrhoids are often troublesome, and can usually be controlled by regulation of the bowels, warm baths, and perhaps anæsthetic ointments, astringent suppositories or compresses of lead lotion. Not infrequently a small perianal thrombosis occurs, causing a tense and acutely painful swelling at the anal margin. It is usually necessary to infiltrate the base of the hæmatoma with lignocaine, incise the swelling and evacuate the clot. This small operation gives dramatic relief, and no post-operative treatment is required except local cleanliness and baths twice a day. If, after delivery, piles require treatment, the patient is sent to a rectal surgeon, but usually piles regress and seldom require operation.

PRURITUS

Irritation of the vulva is often associated with thrush, and testing the urine for sugar is always indicated. Treatment is along the lines indicated on p. 146. Local congestion and vulval varices are other causes of pruritus, which will cease spontaneously after delivery.

VAGINAL DISCHARGE

A slight increase in the normal vaginal secretion is common, and the anxiety many patients feel can be dispelled. It is necessary, however, to ensure that it is not due to a vaginal infection such as thrush (p. 140).

ŒDEMA

Œdema in pregnant patients should always be regarded as a

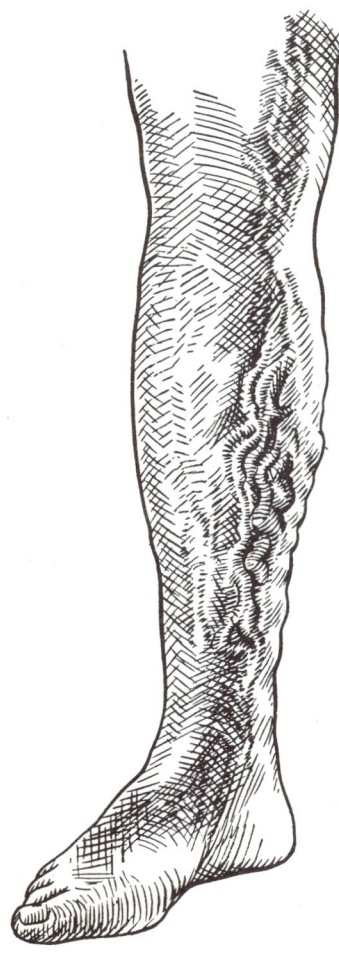

FIG. 99. Varicose veins. The whole of the internal saphenous system of veins is dilated.

grave symptom indicating pre-eclamptic toxæmia of pregnancy (p. 218) until this diagnosis has been carefully excluded. Congestive heart failure and chronic nephritis are two conditions that may be responsible, and twin pregnancy is another cause to be considered. At no time of pregnancy should œdema of the dependent parts be considered normal, but there are some patients, especially those with varicose veins, in whom no cause can be found, and rest with the feet up is the most useful treatment for the uncomplicated condition.

INSOMNIA

Some women suffer from sleeplessness during pregnancy, and the usual causes are overt or concealed anxiety, cramps, or disturbance by fetal movements. Adequate antenatal care should help the first, and a mild sedative is best for the second.

BACKACHE

Pain in the back is due partly to stretching of ligaments and partly to the posture that pregnant women adopt, hollowing the back and drawing back the shoulders to balance the weight of the fœtus. Lessons in walking from the physiotherapist, sensible shoes, adequate rest and perhaps mild analgesia should control this symptom.

CONSTIPATION

This is a very common complaint, especially in the early months and will be most troublesome in those whose bowels are not normally very active. Plenty of roughage in the diet and an increased fluid intake are helpful and an aperient such as Senokot is usually necessary. Liquid paraffin is best avoided, since there is some evidence that it interferes with vitamin absorption from the intestine.

MAJOR DISORDERS OF PREGNANCY

EXCESSIVE VOMITING (HYPEREMESIS GRAVIDARUM)

Vomiting in the early months may be so severe as to result in dehydration and ketosis, the appearance of acetone in the urine and in the breath. Some patients are tense and the inferior vena cava, and the glucose administered by caval drip. Infusion of glucose of the strength required into a superficial vein causes thrombosis.

A constant check is kept on the blood chemistry, and if the urinary output is inadequate, and the levels of the blood urea and potassium are rising, treatment by peritoneal dialysis should be begun. This enables water and electrolytes to be removed from the circulation, and so to preserve the patient's life until kidney function recovers. Most patients will recover if they survive until the establishment of diuresis, and peritoneal dialysis is a comparatively simple procedure that can be performed in any hospital. The nurse's duties are largely the maintenance of a sterile technique to prevent peritonitis; accurate recording of the fluid balance, blood pressure and pulse; and watching for clinically significant signs such as fever or low blood pressure that must be reported at once. The doctor is responsible for ordering the correct dialysing fluid, in the light of the findings on the blood chemistry. The question of hæmodialysis with an artificial kidney only arises exceptionally, when the kidneys fail to resume their function.

DIALYSIS

There are two ways in which this can be accomplished. In *hæmodialysis*, blood is taken from an artery (such as the radial artery) through a polythene tube into an artificial kidney machine, in which the blood is only separated by a semipermeable membrane from a layer of dialysing fluid, into which water, urea and salts will pass by a process of diffusion. The blood is returned into a vein, and the process continues for about fourteen hours. The apparatus is complicated, so that hæmodialysis is only performed at special centres.

The second method makes use of the peritoneum as a dialysing membrane, and since it provides an area greater than that of the glomeruli in the kidneys, it is an effective one. The principle is to run fluid of prepared constituents into the peritoneal cavity, allow it to remain there while water and salts diffuse into it from the tissues, and then run it out again and repeat the process. The apparatus is simple and easily set up, the nurse's duties are not complicated, though the estimations of the blood electrolytes that

222 MODERN GYNÆCOLOGY FOR NURSES

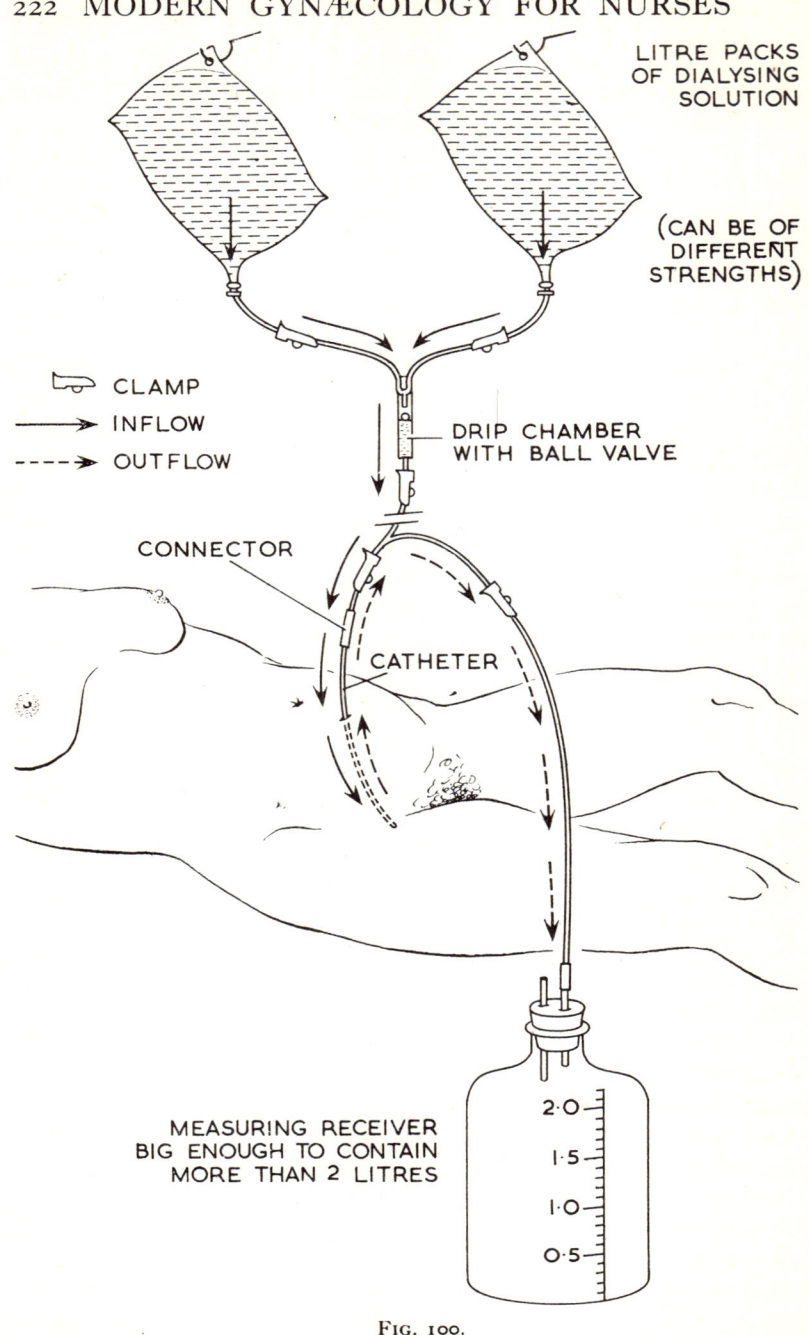

FIG. 100.

enable the doctor to decide what strength of fluid to use are of critical importance. Peritoneal dialysis can be carried out in any hospital where these can be made.

Sterilized disposable apparatus and solutions are prepared by several firms. That described here is Diaflex, by Allen and Hanbury. The solutions used are dispensed in collapsible plastic bags each containing a litre. These must be hypertonic, in order to draw fluid out of the tissues, and two strengths are supplied. The weaker contains 13·6 G of dextrose per litre, and the other, which is used for œdematous patients, contains 63·6 G. Solutions as strong as this can withdraw large amounts of fluid and when they are used constant watch must be kept on the pulse and blood pressure so that the threat of shock can be detected early.

The patient is told about the procedure, and the benefits it will bring. A sedative may be given if she is apprehensive. It is most important that the bladder is empty before dialysis. The patient lies on her back, and the skin is anæsthetized in the midline, about the junction of the upper third and lower two thirds of this line. The skin is nicked with a scalpel, and a trocar and cannula introduced into the peritoneal cavity. The trocar is removed, and the Diaflex catheter passed through it, downwards into the right or left iliac fossa. This catheter has a curve to facilitate its placing, and multiple perforations at the distal end. Prevention of infection is of prime importance, and every aseptic precaution must be taken while the catheter is introduced, and throughout dialysis.

Two bags of fluid are used, warmed to body temperature, and attached to the giving set, which is illustrated in Fig. 100. Clamps on the tubing allow the fluid to be directed from the bags into the abdomen, or from the abdomen into the outflow bag or jar. The process of running the fluid in and out again is termed a cycle, and the amount and rate of giving varies slightly according to the doctor's views. A typical routine is to run a litre in in about twenty minutes, shut the clamps and allow it to remain in the peritoneal cavity for about twenty minutes and then let it run out. By this method, a cycle takes about an hour, and about twelve cycles are given at a time. 500 units of heparin are usually given via the tubing every third cycle, in order to prevent blockage of the catheter holes by fibrin.

Antibiotics are not given as a routine, but the outflow is cultured daily and a gentian violet dressing is applied round the abdominal catheter. Resistance to infection is low in renal failure, and every precaution must be taken. The nurse's observations include:—

(1) *The fluid balance.* If more fluid returns than is run in, this represents a gain from the patient, and is recorded as a minus quantity. The patient is allowed moderate amounts to drink; for instance, the volume of any urine passed, plus 500 ml.

(2) *The temperature*; a rise will indicate infection of the puncture wound or the peritoneum.

(3) *The pulse*; a fall in the volume may indicate shock and must be reported at once. A rising rate again may indicate infection.

(4) *The blood pressure*; a fall is a serious sign, especially if the outflow is much greater than the input, as it indicates that the patient is becoming dehydrated.

Difficulties that may arise in connection with peritoneal dialysis can usually be dealt with quite easily. Pain, especially as the cycle ends, is treated by 5 ml. of lignocaine through the catheter, and usually disappears when the next input starts. Failure of fluid to run out can generally be cured by running more in, or changing the patient's position, but sometimes the catheter must be resited.

Regular estimation is made of the blood electrolytes, especially of potassium, which must be given in doses regulated by the levels in the patient's blood. In many cases, urine secretion is re-established and the patient recovers. If the kidneys are permanently damaged, long term plans must be made, which may include hæmodialysis.

ANTE-PARTUM HÆMORRHAGE

Bleeding from the genital tract before the twenty-eighth week of pregnancy and, therefore, before the fœtus is viable, indicates a threatened abortion (p. 230). Bleeding after the twenty-eighth week is called ante-partum hæmorrhage. It is important not only because it is dangerous to the mother, but also because it indicates that the placenta is being separated from the wall of the uterus and, therefore, the baby's oxygen supply is being reduced or cut off. There are three types of ante-partum hæmorrhage: (i) Unavoidable hæmorrhage; (ii) accidental hæmorrhage, and (iii) incidental hæmorrhage.

Unavoidable Hæmorrhage. This is bleeding that occurs from the site of a placenta which is situated partly or entirely in the lower uterine segment. Such a condition is known as placenta prævia (p. 199). Bleeding from a placenta prævia is called " unavoidable " because, during the formation of the lower uterine segment in the later stages of pregnancy or during labour itself, bleeding from a placenta prævia must occur and cannot be avoided. A patient usually bleeds for the first time at about the thirty-fourth week of pregnancy but bleeding may not occur until she actually commences labour. The bleeding is painless and there is no evidence of pre-eclamptic toxæmia. The bleeding at first is slight in amount and then gradually increases in severity.

Treatment. Although the amount lost may not be great, the patient is kept at rest in bed and the doctor called. A serial record of the pulse and blood pressure should be made until he arrives. An accurate record must be made of the amount of blood lost and all pads and stained garments must be saved for his inspection. The patient receives sedation, probably morphine 16 mgm., and is sent to hospital where she will probably remain until she is delivered. In hospital, blood is taken for hæmoglobin, blood-grouping and cross-matching. A record is kept of the pulse, blood pressure, fetal heart rate and uterine contractions or lack of them. She is treated with complete bed rest and sedation until the bleeding ceases. Then a careful assessment must be made to exclude placenta prævia. A vaginal examination is likely to increase the bleeding, especially in placenta prævia, and should not be undertaken except in hospital and only then in the operating theatre where a Cæsarean section can speedily be performed, if required.

An X-ray is occasionally helpful and failure of the head to descend into the pelvis in a primigravida after the thirty-sixth week suggests that the placenta is low-lying.

Accidental Hæmorrhage. This is hæmorrhage from a placenta that is normally situated in the upper part of the uterus. It may be concealed or revealed, or both. In concealed accidental ante-partum hæmorrhage, the blood does not escape from the uterus but remains within it. If the bleeding becomes more severe or when uterine contractions commence, some of the blood will seep down the uterus, pass through the cervix and will then be revealed. There are many causes of accidental ante-partum hæmorrhage but probably the most common is pre-eclamptic toxæmia. Rarely, trauma may also separate the placenta and cause this type of hæmorrhage. The patient experiences severe abdominal pain and shows such signs of internal bleeding as pallor, sweating, air hunger and a pulse of diminishing volume. The blood pressure may be misleading since it is usually high to begin with. The patient may have hypertension, albuminuria and œdema because she is suffering from pre-eclamptic toxæmia. The uterus is tender and irritable and, in severe instances, is hard and extremely painful (woody uterus). The fetal heart cannot usually be heard.

Treatment. The treatment consists of rest in bed, sedation with morphine 16 mgm., blood transfusion and observation of the pulse, blood pressure and uterine contractions or lack of them. As uterine function returns, blood is lost from the vagina and uterine contractions can be felt through the abdominal walls. Surgical induction of labour can then be performed and delivery of the fetus (which is dead), the placenta and the blood clot, is usually uneventful.

Incidental Hæmorrhage. Incidental hæmorrhage is bleeding from the genital tract from lesions which are incidental to the pregnancy, such as cervical erosions or cervical polypi. Bleeding from these causes is slight.

SPECIAL INVESTIGATIONS IN PREGNANCY

Sound waves up to 20,000 cycles per second are audible to the human ear. Waves of still higher frequency (about 2·5 million cycles per second) are inaudible, but have a variety of uses in medicine. Some of these are curative, some are diagnostic, just as X-rays are, and it is the latter which are important in differentiating between normal and some abnormal states in pregnancy and conditions from which it may have to be diagnosed. No harm to the fetus has been traced to the use of ultrasonics, whereas X-rays carry some risk.

Several types of machine are in use. Some are used to show the position of the pelvic structures by means of a sonar scan. Conditions such as ovarian cyst, uterine fibroids and incomplete abortion can be shown, and ultrasound is the best way of demonstrating the hydatidiform mole mentioned above. Later in pregnancy such conditions as multiple fetuses or hydrocephalus can be shown, and a good estimate of the expected date of delivery can be made by measuring the fetal head. The nurse should notice that unlike other gynæcological examinations, this one requires that the bladder should be full.

Another type of machine produces a result within the audible range, which can be heard through a loud speaker. The fetal heart can be heard by the twelfth week or soon after by this machine, and it can also be used during labour to monitor the fetal heart, and give early warning of fetal distress.

CHAPTER 13
ABORTION

AFTER the twenty-eighth week of pregnancy, the fetus is capable of independent existence, though its chances of survival if labour occurs so early are not great. Expulsion of the fetus from the uterus before the twenty-eighth week is termed abortion or miscarriage, the two terms being synonymous.

The actual number of pregnancies that end in abortion cannot be known exactly, since a number never receive any medical care, but most surgeons believe that one in five of all pregnancies result in abortion.

Abortion is now legal in this country, providing certain criteria are fulfilled and a certificate is signed by two doctors.

The indications for procuring an abortion are:—

(1) If continuation of the pregnancy would endanger the life or health of the mother to a greater extent than its termination.

(2) If there is a reasonable chance that the baby will be severely deformed.

(3) If the continuation of the pregnancy is going to have a harmful effect upon the children of the marriage.

Any abortion must be performed in a National Health Service hospital, or in an authorized institution. In the first half of 1973, there were 57,490 abortions, a rise of 6% on the year before. Those surgeons who have religious or moral objections to abortion are of course entitled to observe these.

CAUSES OF ABORTION

Often the cause of abortion cannot be ascertained, but the following are among the reasons known.

Maternal

(1) General diseases like hypertension or chronic heart disease.

(2) Any acute febrile condition such as the specific fevers.

(3) Endocrine dysfunction, such as thyrotoxicosis or diabetes. Deficiency of the corpus luteum secretion, which is necessary for the maintenance of pregnancy, has been postulated.

(4) Local conditions such as underdevelopment of the uterus, fibroids, or congenital abnormalities of the uterus.

Fetal

(1) Blighted ovum. This is a pregnancy in which the chorion and amniotic sac are normal, but the fœtus does not develop. It is considered by many obstetricians to be one of the commonest causes of spontaneous abortion.

(2) Fetal abnormalities are a common cause of abortion.

(3) Abnormal implantation of the fetus in the uterus, e.g., attachment of the placenta near the internal os.

Criminal

Not only unmarried girls who have become pregnant, but married women who already have large families, may endeavour to terminate their pregnancies themselves or resort to an abortionist. Since the interference is made without aseptic precautions and without an anæsthetic, the results are often disastrous. Endometritis and even peritonitis occur, hæmorrhage may be severe, and sudden death from shock or air embolism is not infrequently reported. So is perforation of the vagina, bladder or uterus.

Nurses are reminded that such operations are illegal, as well as highly dangerous. If asked to assist with the treatment of a woman who is bleeding, they should undertake no procedures without the instructions of a doctor. If their advice is sought about the possibility of procuring abortion, they should refer the patient to her own doctor, so that the pregnancy can be terminated according to the Abortion Act, if the necessary criteria are fulfilled.

SIGNS AND SYMPTOMS OF ABORTION

Most abortions occur in the first three months of pregnancy, before the maturity of the placenta, and the detachment of the ovum is accompanied by bleeding which can be very profuse. Loss of this kind is accompanied by painful contractions of the uterus, dilation of the cervix and expulsion of the ovum and its membranes. Slight, or even moderate, bleeding does not, however, mean that the pregnancy must end.

Several varieties of abortion are encountered clinically.

(1) Threatened Abortion. The patient, who is in the early stages of pregnancy, is losing a little blood per vaginam. She may have some abdominal discomfort but no actual pain, because rhythmic uterine contractions are not present. Vaginal examination is not usually done at this stage for fear of increasing the uterine disturbance, but if it is, the cervix will be closed.

The patient is put to bed with one or two pillows, and if she has some pain and is alarmed (and most patients who come to hospital at this stage are anxious to preserve their pregnancy) morphine 10 mgm. is given. Some surgeons use progesterone or œstrogen, though many are not convinced that hormones are useful.

Pads must be saved, and any increase in bleeding or pain reported. A low residue diet is given, and aperients, and above all enemata, avoided. Phenobarbitone 60 mgm. b.d. is often prescribed for a nervous patient. She should stay in bed for three days after the bleeding stops, and then should avoid physical or mental stress until the pregnancy is well established. Coitus is forbidden.

(2) Inevitable Abortion. Bleeding may continue and rhythmic uterine contractions occur. If the cervix dilates, or any portion of the fœtal membranes is passed, abortion is inevitable. It should be hastened only if blood loss is excessive, by the administration of an intramuscular injection of ergometrine mgm. 0·5, if bleeding does not cease soon after the expulsion of the products of conception. An intramuscular injection of ergometrine 0·5 mgm. will be ordered to stimulate the uterine contractions and stop the hæmorrhage. Anything passed per vaginam must be saved for inspection, as it is important to know if all the products of conception have been expelled. Following the abortion, the thighs should be washed with soap and water, the vulva swabbed and dried, and a sterile pad applied. Subsequently the nurse assures herself that bleeding is slight. The vulva is swabbed twice a day, and when no more bright blood is being lost, and if the temperature is normal, the patient may go home. This is usually on the third day.

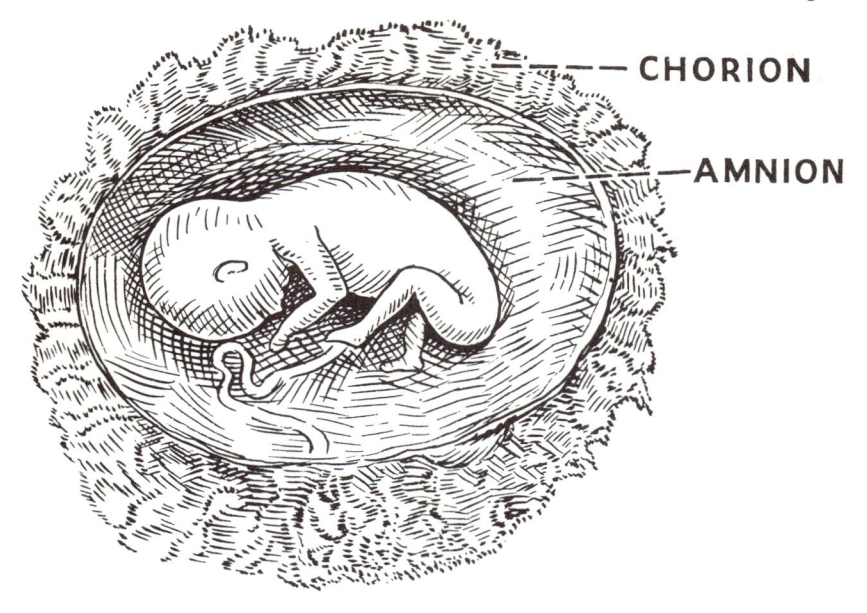

FIG. 101. Complete abortion. The fetus and its membranes may be passed intact. In this diagram the anterior portion of the chorion has been removed.

(3) Complete Abortion. It is hoped that every inevitable abortion will end as a complete one, i.e., that the uterus is emptied. Sometimes, however, portions of the fetal membranes are retained, and the case then falls into the next category.

(4) Incomplete Abortion. Portions of the products of conception may remain in the uterus when the fetus is passed. Bleeding may be severe, or may be slight but continuous. The patient should have the uterus evacuated surgically under a general anæsthetic.

(5) Missed Abortion. Cases occur in which abortion is threatened, but the bleeding ceases and all is apparently well. The signs of pregnancy, however, subside; breast activity ceases, and the uterus does not enlarge. A brownish discharge begins, after an interval, from the uterus, and indicates that the ovum is dead, but retained in utero. It degenerates into a solid mass, mostly of organised blood clot called a CARNEOUS MOLE.

This will in time be expelled with little or no loss, and may be hastened by the administration of ergot by mouth, and of stilbœstrol. Surgical evacuation of the uterus may become necessary if the process is long delayed.

(6) **Septic Abortion.** Sepsis may supervene after any abortion, especially if it is incomplete or the result of criminal interference. The temperature is high, the abdomen tender in the lower part, and bright blood continues to be lost, while this discharge may become offensive.

Penicillin may be begun at once, as the infection is often streptococcal, and a cervical swab sent for a report on the sensitivity of the organism to antibiotics. If the abortion is incomplete, evacuation of the uterus can be undertaken in the theatre, once the infection has been controlled. Afterwards antibiotics will be continued, a high fluid intake encouraged, and regular vulval toilet instituted.

After any abortion, a large area within the uterus is open to infection, and salpingitis may occur as the result of an ascending infection, and cause much chronic ill-health. An abortion should always be considered to carry the risk of uterine sepsis or its pelvic complications.

(7) **Habitual abortion.** This term implies that abortion has occurred three or more times, at about the same stage of pregnancy, and is thought to have the same cause on each occasion. There are many causes, functional and anatomical, and in some cases no cause can be identified. There may be congenitally small uterus, or a structural abnormality, or uterine fibroids, and if the condition is amenable to surgery, an operation is performed. Sometimes it is thought that the cervix is not competent to retain the growing fetus, and for such women a pursestring suture may be inserted around the cervix. This stitch is removed at term, or when labour begins.

METHODS OF THERAPEUTIC ABORTION

The methods by which abortion is induced are always changing, and better, safer and speedier techniques are constantly being tested. However, there is no branch of work in which it is more important to remember that this is a situation in which the interests of the patient are the prime consideration. Once it has been decided that termination is indicated, and that the patient fully concurs, abortion is undertaken by the method most appropriate to her and to the duration of her pregnancy. Since this is a book for nurses, it must also be mentioned that many nurses find problems in adjusting to the care of women undergoing abortion, since the termination of fetal life arouses feelings of anxiety even in those who do not have religious objections. Senior nurses must be aware of the need to guide juniors to accept fully a medical decision which is judged to be in the woman's best interests, and to guard against inadvertently displaying any signs of a judgmental attitude. All patients whose pregnancy has been terminated must receive good and suitable contraceptive advice, but even so some will return for a second termination. It often seems that there is a deeper reason than heedlessness for recurring pregnancy, and the psychologist may say that the woman feels an unspoken need for motherhood, even if it is socially inconvenient. She may ask strange questions, such as "Will it hurt the baby?", and in such circumstances the nurse should seek the guidance of a perceptive senior.

The following methods of terminating pregnancy are arranged approximately in chronological order of availability.

(1) The "morning after" pill. Large doses of stilbœstrol can be given by mouth in the very early days after a period has been missed in a woman previously regular. Careful follow-up is necessary, because if this method fails, the pregnancy must be terminated in another way, because there is a risk of vaginal neoplasm in a female fetus of which the mother has received such large doses of stilbœstrol.

(2) Menstrual extraction. This is again a method that can be used soon after a missed period. General anæsthesia is not required, and this is an out-patient procedure. With the patient in the lithotomy position, a narrow plastic cannula is passed through the cervix and suction applied. The possibility of rupturing a uterus softened by early pregnancy must be remembered.

(3) Dilatation and curettage of uterus can be performed

in the theatre under general anæsthesia. It is best undertaken before the twelfth week of pregnancy.

(4) Suction termination is quite commonly used, again with a general anæsthetic. A stainless steel catheter is used, and suction of about 400 mm. of mercury.

(5) Prostaglandin administration. These substances were originally identified in semen, and it was thought they derived from the prostate. In fact, they come from the seminal vesicles, and from many other tissues too. They are mediators of inflammation, there are many naturally occurring and synthetic forms, and because they stimulate uterine contraction they are used in the termination of pregnancy and the induction of labour. Prostaglandins may be administered as vaginal pessaries or by injection directly into the uterus. They may be given intravenously together with oxytocin. This method can be used up to the 18th week, and usually results in expulsion of conception products within twelve hours. Nausea and vomiting may occur. Analgesics can be given in full dosage, as the well-being of the fetus does not have to be considered. The process is like a miniature labour, and is a trying experience for a woman, especially if she has told no one of the termination, and so is alone. It can of course also be stressful for staff.

6. Various substances such as concentrated saline can be introduced into the amniotic sac to induce abortion.

7. Hysterotomy by the abdominal route can be undertaken if the pregnancy is further advanced. The preparation and aftercare is as for any other abdominal operation.

8. Intravenous oxytocin (Syntocinon) infusion. The amount is gradually increased until regular uterine contractions are established, and infusion is usually continued until one hour after abortion, in order to minimize bleeding.

Careful follow-up is essential after abortion, since some morbidity occurs even under the best conditions. The further advanced the pregnancy, the higher is the incidence of complications.

VESICULAR OR HYDATIDIFORM MOLE

This curious condition is produced by a degeneration of the chorion, which occurs about the second month of pregnancy and causes death of the fetus. The chorion is converted into a mass of small cysts, often growing at a rapid

ABORTION

rate. Cases are seen at all ages, but a considerable number are women over forty.

The patient has usually missed one or two periods, and often experiences severe morning sickness, with headache, œdema of the ankles, and sometimes albuminuria. Intermittent bloodstained discharge occurs, and bleeding may become continuous. When she is examined, the uterus is enlarged much beyond the expected size, but neither palpation nor X-ray reveals a fetus, though pregnancy tests are strongly positive at dilutions of greater than 1 in 200.

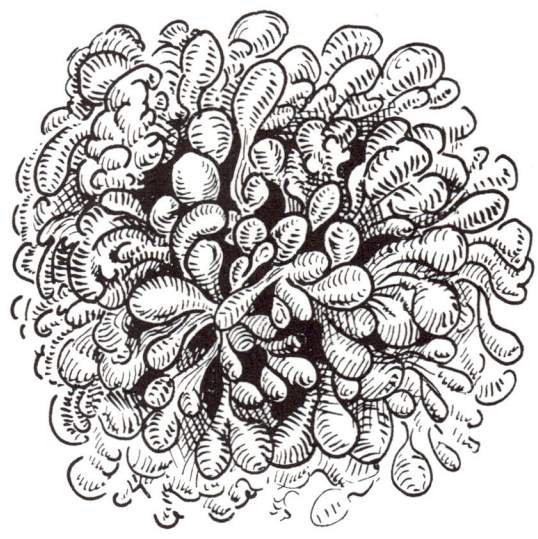

FIG. 102. Hydatidiform or Vesicular Mole.

The complications of a vesicular or hydatidiform mole are:—
(1) Hæmorrhage when the mole is expelled or removed.
(2) Sepsis.
(3) Malignancy.

Treatment

It is usually necessary to evacuate the uterus surgically, though sometimes the mole is expelled spontaneously. Under a general anæsthetic the cervix is slowly dilated and the mole removed manually. Ergometrine 0·5 mgm. or oxytocin 5 units is given intravenously to contract the uterus and minimize bleeding. Regular vulval toilet is performed following evacuation, and since a large area in the uterus is left raw, a prophylactic course of penicillin may be ordered. The patient should not leave hospital until bleeding has ceased, and careful follow-up is imperative because of the risk of appearance of an exceedingly malignant condition, chorion epithelioma, or choriocarcinoma.

CHORION EPITHELIOMA

Since this type of cancer arises from the chorion, it can only develop after pregnancy. It may follow abortion or a full-term pregnancy, but 40% of the recorded cases have followed a vesicular mole.

A diagnostic feature of this condition is that pregnancy tests become strongly positive again, so that such a test should be performed three and nine weeks after evacuation of a vesicular mole, and then every six months for two years, and the patient should be told to report at once any discharge or abnormal bleeding, which would indicate the necessity for a diagnostic curettage. The patient must be kept under observation for two years.

If chorion epithelioma occurs, the pregnancy test becomes strongly positive, and bleeding begins. The growth soon infiltrates the uterus and vagina, and pain and cachexia occur. Spread by the bloodstream is common, especially to the lungs. This is one of the most rapidly fatal growths in women.

Treatment is by total hysterectomy and removal of the tubes and ovaries as soon as the diagnosis is made. Cases have been recorded in which metastases in the lungs have disappeared following the removal of the primary. Deep X-ray therapy may be tried, since some chorion epitheliomata are remarkably radio-sensitive. Methotrexate, one of the cytotoxic drugs, is very effective against the metastases, and is the treatment of choice.

CHAPTER 14

LABOUR AND DELIVERY

THE factor that determines the onset of labour is not precisely known, though it is believed that the pituitary, whose hormone pitocin causes contraction of uterine muscle, is probably responsible. During the later weeks of pregnancy, a hand placed on the abdomen will detect painless contractions of the uterus fifteen to twenty times a minute. At term these contractions, hitherto painless, become regular and painful, and labour has begun.

Three well-marked stages occur in labour.

(1) The first stage is the longest, and lasts from the onset of labour to full dilatation of the cervix. Before labour begins the cervical canal measures about 2·5 cm. in length. When labour starts, the cervix opens a little (enough in a primigravida to admit one finger), and no further dilatation takes place until the length of the cervical canal has been obliterated by progressive shortening. This is known as "taking up of the cervix." When the cervix is fully taken up, and only then, does dilatation of the cervix continue (see Fig. 103). This stage usually lasts eighteen to twenty-four hours with a first baby, and up to eighteen hours in subsequent pregnancies.

(2) When the cervix is fully dilated, the second stage begins, and lasts until completion of the delivery of the baby. This stage is marked by strong contractions which expel the baby from the uterus into the vagina and thence to the exterior. It may be very short in a multigravida, but usually takes a half to one hour in a first confinement.

(3) The third stage is that in which the placenta is expelled. The time varies, being longer in the case of a first baby, but is usually complete in fifteen minutes.

MANAGEMENT OF THE FIRST STAGE OF LABOUR

When labour begins, the situation of the pain first appreciated by the mother as a labour pain is in the middle of the sacrum, and not at first in the abdomen at all, but soon

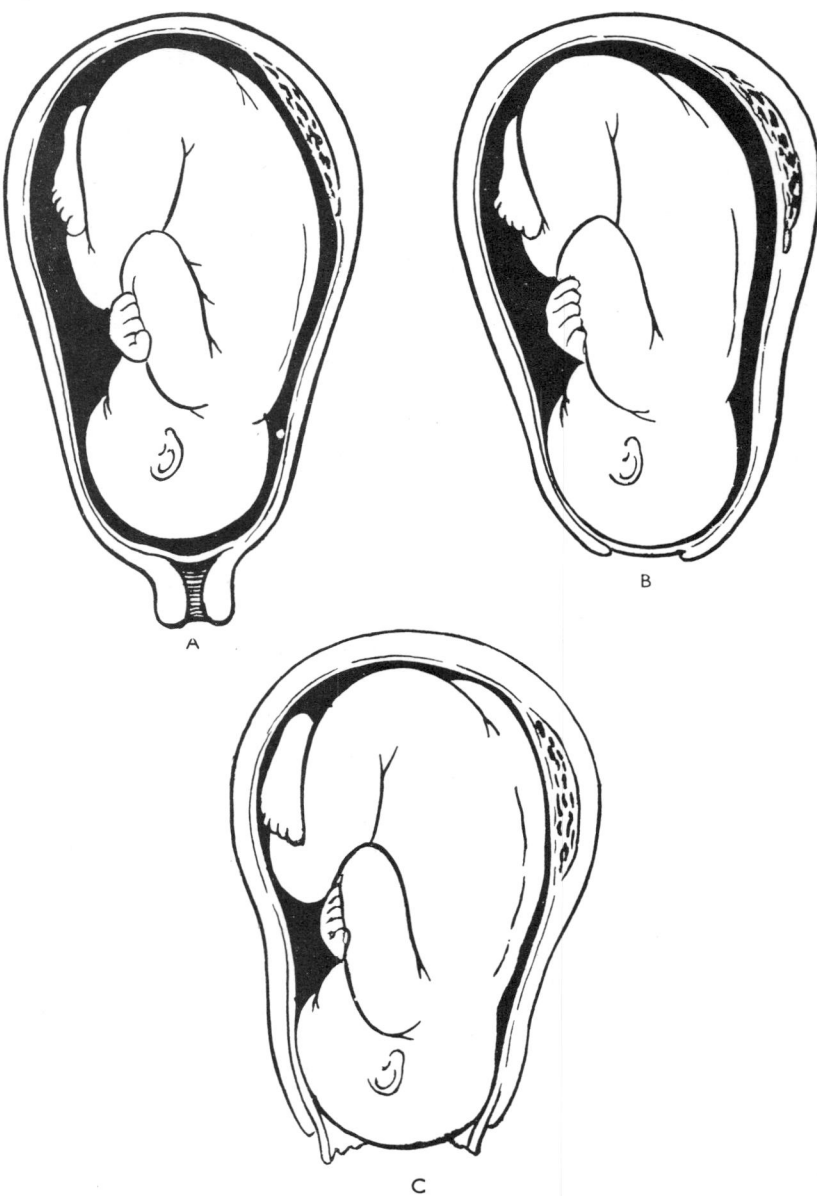

FIG. 103. The first stage of labour.
A. The cervical canal at the onset of labour.
B. The cervix has been taken up and the os is dilating.
C. The cervix is fully dilated, the membranes have ruptured, and the second stage of labour begins.

it begins to travel round to the front. At the same time that regular painful contractions are established, the mucus that has blocked the cervical canal during pregnancy is dislodged, and is passed together with a little blood. This constitutes the " show," and is additional evidence that labour has begun.

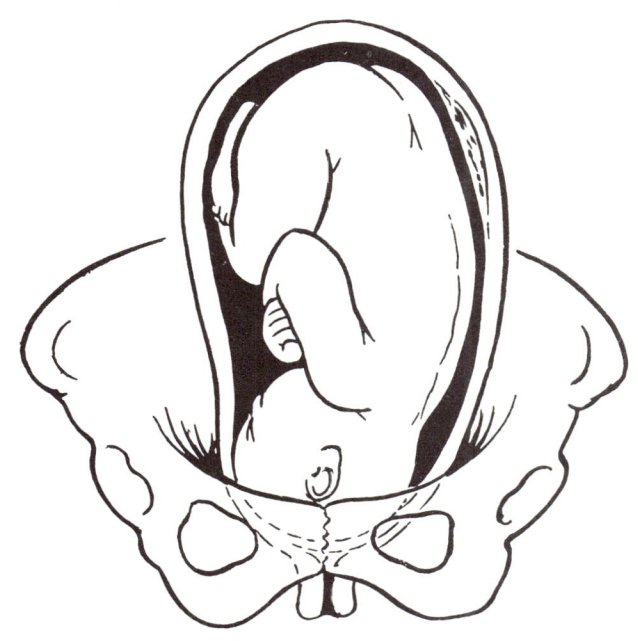

Fig. 104. Vertex presentation. The head lies obliquely in the pelvis, with the occiput in front and to the left. This is the most common presentation.

When the patient arrives in hospital, she is received into the admission room, and is asked what time the pains began, if they are regular, and what is the interval between them. The temperature, pulse, respiration rate and blood pressure are recorded; the ankles and hands are inspected for œdema; a specimen of urine is tested for albumin, sugar and acetone; and the patient is seen and examined by a midwife or doctor.

The abdomen is palpated to find how the baby is presenting, and in the normal case the head will be engaged in the pelvis, lying in the oblique diameter with the occiput to the front, so that the baby's back can be felt through the abdominal wall, half turned to the left or right. The fetal heart can be heard beating, and often during examination the uterus will be felt to harden, and the patient says a pain is beginning.

The bladder is emptied, and a specimen of urine examined for the common abnormalities, and for ketones. A full bladder may be injured in the second stage, especially if this is long and the baby a big one. Distension of the bladder also inhibits contraction of the uterus during all stages of labour, and the nurse sees to it that such distension does not occur.

The pubis and vulva are shaved, and if the membranes are intact and labour not too far advanced, an enema is given, since a loaded rectum delays labour and complicates delivery. A bath, or preferably a shower, is given, the nurse remaining with her patient, who is then put to bed.

The mother-to-be has many physical needs, which are described below. Above all, however, she looks to the nurse for reassurance and comfort. There lie ahead some hours of discomfort, during which the patient can make no contribution yet towards the baby's birth. She needs company, and should not be left alone for more than short periods; if the husband is available, he should be allowed to stay with his wife. Patients left alone worry about the increasing severity and frequency of the pains, the meaning of the escape of liquor, or whether the baby may be born unexpectedly with no one at hand. Every time an examination is made, or the fetal heart auscultated, the patient is told that all is well. Tension and fear not only prolong labour by inhibiting uterine contractions, but also predispose to bleeding afterwards.

Vaginal examinations are performed only when necessary, since even with a meticulous technique there is a risk of infecting the birth canal. The patient should be well washed with soap and water from the hips to the knees beforehand, and the vulva swabbed with such a lotion as hibitane. The operator must be masked, and wear sterile gloves. The information gained may include the following:—

(1) The condition of the vulva and vagina.
(2) The state of the cervix, whether taken up or no.
(3) Whether the cervix is dilated, and if so, how much.
(4) If the membranes are intact.
(5) What is the presenting part of the baby, and how far

LABOUR AND DELIVERY

it has advanced into the pelvis. In most cases it is the head, and effort is made to determine the position by feeling for the sagittal suture and (if the cervix is sufficiently dilated) the posterior fontanelle. Locating this triangular space towards the front of the pelvis is reassuring; the baby's head is well flexed, and therefore presenting its smallest measurement ready for the passage through the pelvis.

(6) The state of the soft tissues of the introitus; if they are rigid they offer resistance to the passage of the baby, and may be torn during delivery if special precautions are not taken.

(7) Whether the rectum is empty.

If labour is established but not too far advanced, an analgesic should be given, since the first stage may be long and tedious, and on the successful management of the patient at this stage will depend her co-operation during delivery. Drugs given to the patient will also affect the baby, and they must be carefully selected. Those used in the first stage include the following:—

(1) Mild sedatives used to allay fear and abolish apprehension. Chloral hydrate is often given as syrup of chloral 10 ml., which contains 2 G. of chloral hydrate. Tranquillizers such as methylpentynol ("Oblivon") 0·25 to 0·5 G. are often given to the nervous patient in early labour.

(2) Analgesics are given to ease or abolish actual pain. The amount of pain felt varies from one woman to another, and bears little relation to the strength of the contractions. An intelligent assessment should be made of the patient's state of mind and the pain she experiences, and the progress of labour must be known accurately. Morphine 10 mgm. is sometimes ordered if contractions are weak and irregular, and the patient very frightened. It must not be given late in the first stage or the baby's respiration centre may be depressed. Pethidine 100 mgm. by intramuscular injection is highly effective. Occasionally tranquillizers are given with pethidine to enhance its action, e.g. Sparine 25 mgm. When the first stage is well advanced nalorphine is given with pethidine (as pethilorphan) to ensure that the pethidine will not depress in any way the respiratory efforts of the newborn baby.

(3) Barbiturates. At night the patient must be encouraged to sleep, or at least to relax completely, in the

intervals between contractions. Or butobarbitone 200 mgm. will ensure good and sound sleep and often the patient will wake in strong labour in the early hours of the morning.

(4) Inhalation analgesics. Towards the end of the first stage and during the second gas and oxygen (see p. 244) is very effective.

The patient can be given fluids if delivery is not expected for some hours, but fluids remain in the stomach for a long time during labour, and care must be taken if an anæsthetic is necessary later. She is encouraged to empty her bladder at intervals. There is no need for her to remain in bed in the early stages, and she may feel more comfortable if she can walk about from time to time.

The records to be kept are:

(1) The temperature, pulse and respiration four-hourly, and the pulse rate more frequently as labour progresses.

(2) The intake and output.

(3) Any drugs given.

(4) The intervals between contractions, and their strength, which can be estimated by a hand on the fundus.

(5) The fetal heart rate, taken between contractions, first two-hourly, then more frequently.

(6) The report of vaginal examination, if the doctor or midwife makes one.

(7) The nature of any vaginal loss. The escape of brown-stained liquor and a rising fetal heart rate indicate fetal distress, and the obstetrician must be informed at once.

(8) The amount of sleep, and the patient's reactions.

During the first stage the uterus is, with each contraction, drawing up the cervix and widening its opening. The cervix does not descend again between contractions, so that each pain means that dilatation increases, until the cervix has been completely drawn up over the head, and the second stage begins.

THE SECOND STAGE

PRESENTATION

Up to the thirty-second week of pregnancy, the fetus has room to move actively within the uterus, but after this date space is no longer available for free movement, and the position of the fetus is stabilized in a longitudinal lie with the head over the brim of the pelvis. This is known as a vertex presentation. The muscle of the uterus tends to keep the fetus in the most compact shape possible—arms and elbows are folded across the chest, and the hips and knees are flexed. The exact reason why the head is usually the lowest part is not known but it may be because it is the heaviest. The long axis of the head lies diagonally across the pelvis, with the occiput towards the front. This occipito-anterior position is the normal and also the most favourable presentation, the left being slightly more common than the right. The head should be well flexed in order to present its smallest diameter to the pelvic brim, just as one flexes the head in order to pull on a tight sweater.

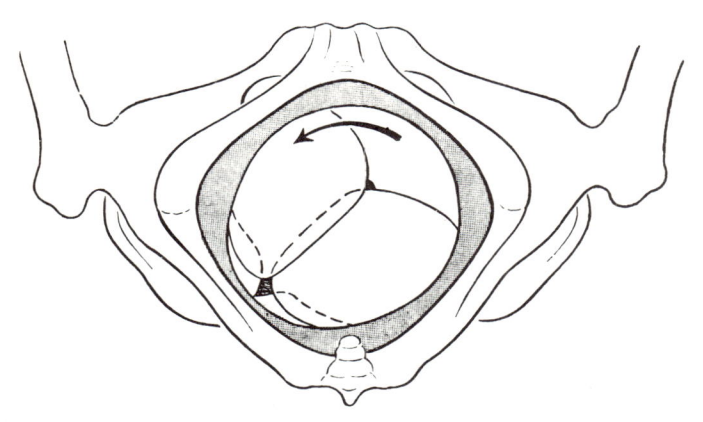

FIG. 105. The female pelvis. A view from below, showing the position of the baby's head in the left occipito-anterior presentation, and the direction of rotation.

The commonest abnormality of presentation is that the occiput is posterior, i.e. lies to the right or left of the sacrum. The main disadvantages of such a position are that the first stage is often prolonged, painful and tedious because the head has a long way to rotate to bring the occiput to the front; that instrumental delivery is often required; and that bleeding in the third stage is rather more common because of the long first stage. The prolonged labour demands skill, sympathy and vigilance from the midwife.

When the buttocks are the lowest part, the baby is said to present by the breech. The risks to the child of a breech presentation are not inconsiderable and one of the aims of antenatal care is to detect such a position and, if possible, to correct it by turning the baby. There are two dangers to the baby that presents by the breech: (*a*) breathing may be attempted before the head has been delivered from the vagina; (*b*) over-rapid delivery of the head may result in tears of the tentorium, the fold of meninges that separates cerebrum and cerebellum. It will be seen that the second stage must be conducted briskly enough to avoid asphyxia and slowly enough to avoid cerebral damage and such skill is one of the arts of midwifery.

Other malpresentations are uncommon and need not be considered in this context.

ANALGESIA IN THE SECOND STAGE

Although relatively short, the second stage of labour is painful to most women, especially when the perineum is being stretched by the advancing head. Some inhalational analgesic is usually given, and suitable ones must satisfy two criteria. They must be safe both for mother and baby, and must be effective without interfering with consciousness to such an extent that the mother cannot co-operate during delivery.

The midwife is, under certain circumstances, allowed to give inhalation analgesics when a doctor is not present. Gas (nitrous oxide) and oxygen may be given, provided that the midwife is experienced and proficient in their use; that the doctor has certified the patient fit to receive them; and that a third person, acceptable to the mother and the midwife, is present.

The usual inhalation analgesic used in the second stage is a mixture of gas (nitrous oxide) and oxygen in equal proportions. This is used by midwives in a pre-mixed cylinder apparatus called Entonox. This mixture has the great advantage over gas and air, which it has superseded, that it maintains full oxygenation of the blood, so that there is no risk to the baby of anoxia from this cause, even if the second stage is prolonged.

EPIDURAL ANALGESIA

The spinal cord is enclosed by the meninges, and around the outer one or dura mater, is the epidural space. This is continuous from the base of the skull to the coccyx, is filled with connective tissue and blood vessels, and is traversed by the spinal nerves on their way to the cord. Local anaesthetics injected into this space, either in the lumbar or caudal regions, will spread to an extent that depends on the volume injected, and on the position of the patient. Since the sensory fibres are rather more susceptible to the anæsthetic than are motor fibres, it is possible to block sensation without undue interference with movement. The patient lies in the left lateral position with the spine flexed, as for lumbar puncture; a special needle is introduced through the anæsthetized skin until its tip lies in the epidural space, a fine polythene catheter is threaded along it, and the needle withdrawn. The catheter is strapped to the patient's back,

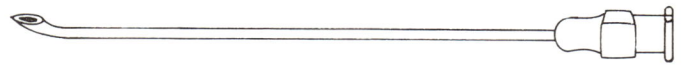

FIG. 106. Epidural needle.

and anæsthetic can be injected as required. Painless labour is possible, though not invariably achieved, and there are no harmful effects on the baby. Epidural anæsthesia requires the presence of an anæsthetist skilled in this technique, so it is not universally available. Where it is, it may be used if a long or difficult labour is anticipated for women with hypertension, and if analgesics are ineffective. Not all women find this kind of analgesic acceptable, and the patient must of course be consulted. The nurse must not leave a patient who has had an epidural injection and should record the blood pressure every two minutes for the first six minutes, and thereafter every fifteen minutes, since hypotension is not uncommon A noticeable fall in the diastolic pressure, especially in the hypertensive, must be at once reported. Bladder difficulties sometimes happen, and the output must be measured.

MANAGEMENT OF THE SECOND STAGE

If delivery is taking place in hospital, the patient is transferred to the labour room when the second stage commences. If the labour ward midwife does not know her she should ascertain her name and call her by it.

The nurse, as this stage approaches, has made her preparations for delivery. A warm cradle is prepared, and the following laid on a trolley, all articles being sterile:—

1 bowl with dry swabs and pads.
1 kidney dish.
3 sterile towels.
Tray with 2 pairs of pressure forceps and scissors.
Tray with a gallipot of normal saline, gauze and wool swabs for the baby's mouth and eyes and 2 cord ligatures.
Covered bin for used dressings.

During the second stage, the baby is pushed by the contracting uterus and by the expulsive efforts of the mother through the fully dilated cervix and vagina, between the levator ani muscles and out through the introitus. Its direction is first backwards, then forwards under the pubic arch. The doctor aims to conduct this stage with the minimum of exhaustion and pain to his patient, without

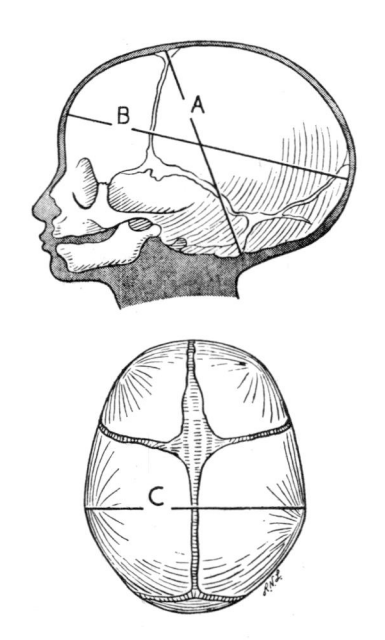

FIG. 107. Fetal skull.

A. Suboccipito-bregmatic, the smallest diameter of the skull.
B. Occipito-frontal diameter.
C. Bi-parietal, the widest diameter of the head.

LABOUR AND DELIVERY

damage to her muscles and perineum, and without risk to the baby.

The membranes will rupture at the beginning of this stage if they have not done so previously, and the liquor escapes. The patient is now encouraged as each pain begins to take several deep breaths of gas and oxygen through the mask, then to hold her breath and bear firmly down. Between pains she should relax as completely as possible.

THE MECHANISM OF LABOUR

The pressure of the fundus of the contracting uterus on the baby's buttocks causes increasing flexion of the spine and neck, so that the head descends on to the forward slope of the pelvic floor, and is directed under the symphysis

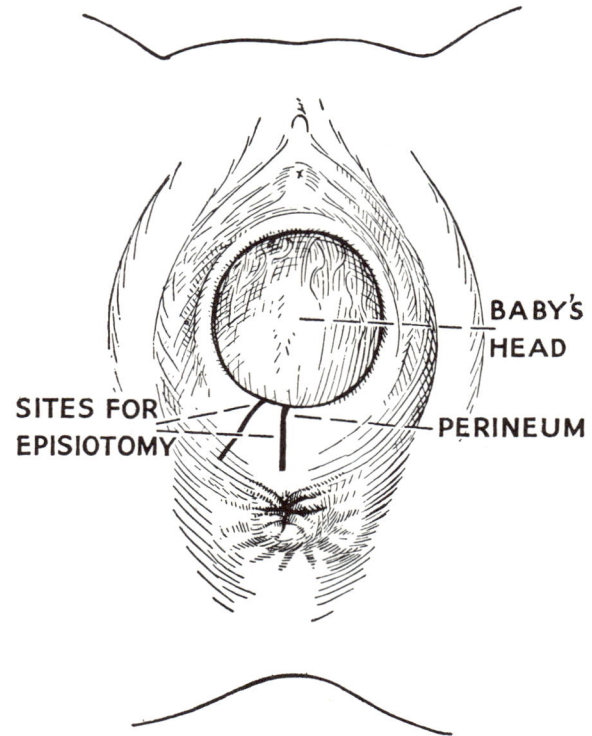

FIG. 108. Episiotomy. In order to avoid a perineal tear, an incision may be made on one of the lines indicated.

pubis. The occiput rotates to the front, and is born beneath the pubic arch. The neck straightens and extends once the broadest diameter of the head has escaped, so that the face appears from beneath the perineum. The head, which had to turn on the shoulders to be born, is now free to rotate back again. The shoulders now turn to lie in the antero-posterior diameter of the pelvis as did the head, and with the next pain the anterior shoulder passes under the pubic arch. The posterior shoulder then emerges from under the perineum, and the trunk and legs are delivered by a movement of lateral flexion, sweeping the trunk up on to the mother's abdomen.

As the head descends, the anus is seen to stretch, the perineum to thin out, and the midwife puts on sterile mask, gown and gloves ready for delivery. If it appears that the perineum will not dilate sufficiently to permit passage of the head without tearing, the doctor may make, with scissors, an incision (episiotomy) in the perineum to one side or other of the midline. The head is delivered between pains, and the nose and mouth at once wiped with swabs. The shoulders follow, one at a time, and the child can then be extracted. It is held up by the feet to drain liquor from the lungs and allow blood to reach the vital centres in the brain, and breathing should begin at once, and usually crying. Particular attention is paid to the infant's airway, and any mucus or liquor is removed by means of a mucus extractor. The mother is told the child's sex and congratulated, and the time is noted.

The establishment of breathing is due to stimulation of the baby's respiratory centre in the medulla by oxygen lack as the placenta begins to separate. The compression of the baby's thorax during delivery, and the impact of the relatively cool external air on its skin are other factors.

The first untoward event of the baby's life may be failure to breathe. In most cases this is only transitory; the nose, mouth and pharynx are sucked out with a mucus extractor, and this stimulus, combined with the clearing of the air passages, is usually enough to start the baby breathing.

In true asphyxia, the baby is limp, livid in colour, and the apex beat is weak. This emergency is most common in prematurity; in babies with cerebral damage, or affected by drugs given to the mother; and in those whose oxygen

LABOUR AND DELIVERY

supply has been diminished by placental disease or detachment, or by pressure on a prolapsed umbilical cord.

Treatment is urgent; if it is delayed the baby may have brain damage if it survives. The air passages are cleared, the cord clamped and cut, and the baby laid on its back with the head slightly extended. A small-sized laryngoscope is passed, the trachea intubated, and oxygen given by intermittent positive pressure not exceeding 40 cm. of water. If maternal drugs are a possible cause, an injection of nalorphine is given into the umbilical vein.

When pulsation ceases in the cord, two pairs of pressure forceps are applied, and the cord divided and tied three or

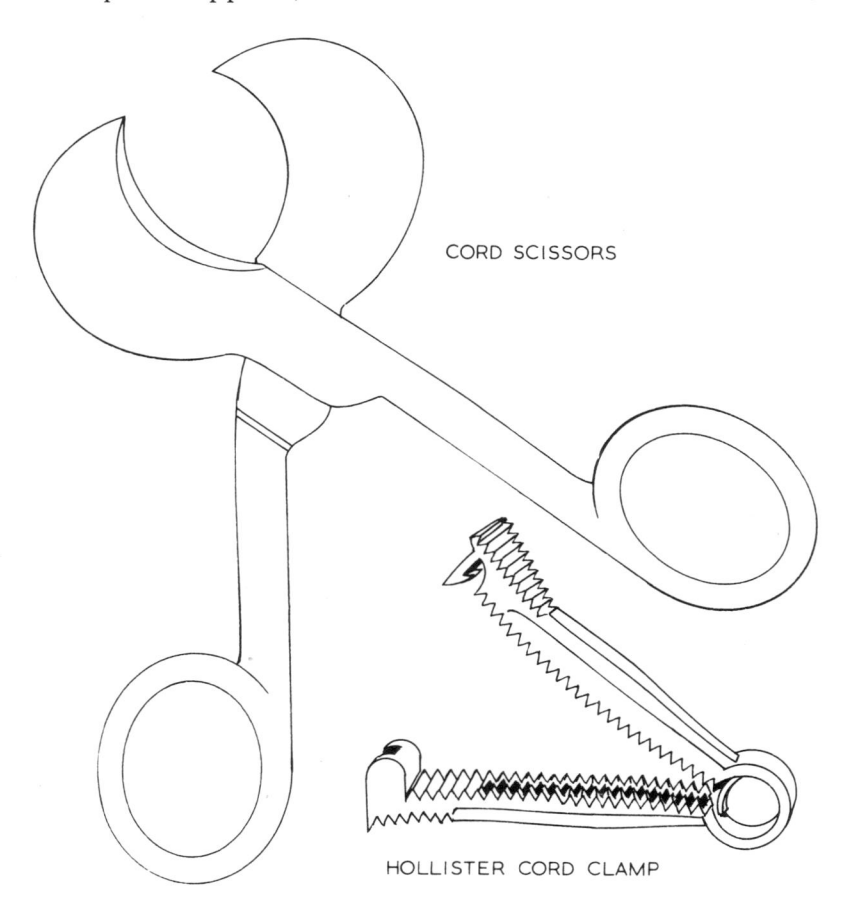

FIG. 109. Hollister clamp.

four inches from the umbilicus. Alternatively, the cord may be compressed with Spencer-Wells forceps and a Hollister disposable clamp applied to the cord, which is then divided flush with the clamp. The baby is wrapped in a sterile towel, may be shown to his mother, and is put in the cradle with the head low, so that mucus and liquor remaining may drain from the air passages. His name should be at once tied to his wrist or ankle, and watch kept that breathing is satisfactory and that no bleeding is taking place from the cord.

THE THIRD STAGE

Meanwhile the mother lies on her back, and a hand on the abdomen will presently reveal that the fundus of the uterus is becoming harder and more elongated as the

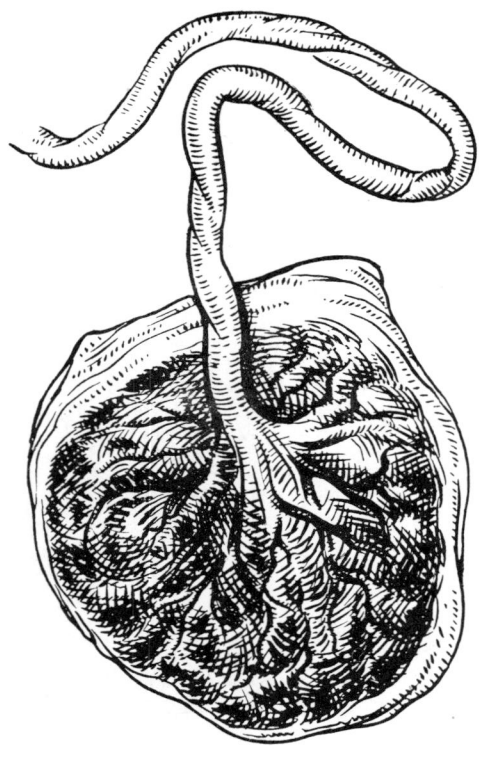

FIG. 110. Placenta. The fetal surface is shown, and the insertion of the cord, and the lobes or cotyledons of which the placenta is made can be seen.

placenta is detached by the contraction of the uterus. It passes into the vagina, whence it is easily expressed into a kidney dish held against the perineum. The placenta is put aside for examination which should show it to be complete; if it is not, steps are taken at once to evacuate the missing portion. The third stage should always be conducted with the patient lying on her back, since in this position the behaviour of the uterus is most easily observed.

If an episiotomy has been performed, or if the perineum has been torn, catgut stitches will now have to be inserted. The pulse rate should be taken, and watch kept that the uterus remains firmly contracted, since poor uterine tone will allow bleeding to occur from the placental site. When she is thought fit, the patient is washed and given clean linen, the vulva is swabbed and dried and a clean sterile pad applied and she is transferred to the lying-in ward.

This brief account is of a typical normal delivery in hospital. The student nurse who works in a maternity ward will know that there are many cases whose course is not so smooth, and that medical, surgical and obstetrical problems may have to be solved. She will realize that a very big field of nursing will be unknown to her unless she takes her midwifery training, and any woman who intends to make nursing her career should, at the end of her training, consider obtaining her midwifery certificate.

THE ACTIVE MANAGEMENT OF LABOUR

Now that so many aids are available to permit, with safety to mother and baby, delivery on a planned date following a shortened labour, the active management of labour is used with increasing frequency. It implies induction of labour, instrumental or assisted delivery if indicated, and shortening of the third stage. The indications may be maternal (e.g. hypertension) or fetal (e.g. post-maturity, Rhesus complications), and increasingly social reasons are acceptable. For instance, the patient may be moving house, and does not want to change obstetricians and the nurses she knows.

INDUCTION OF LABOUR. An intravenous infusion of oxytocin (Syntocinon) in dextrose saline is used to stimulate uterine contractions, the dose and rate being regulated by the effect. Careful monitoring of the duration, amplitude

252 MODERN GYNÆCOLOGY FOR NURSES

and frequency of contractions is needed, and the uterus must be seen to relax between contractions. Analgesics are given in the usual way, and epidural anæsthesia is often selected.

ARTIFICIAL RUPTURE OF MEMBRANES. Integrity of the membranes until the cervix is fully dilated is not seen as vital in the programme of active management as when labour is allowed to run a longer course. When the head is engaged in the pelvis, uterine contractions are regular. The membranes are punctured with amniotomy forceps and when the cervix is dilated about 3cm.

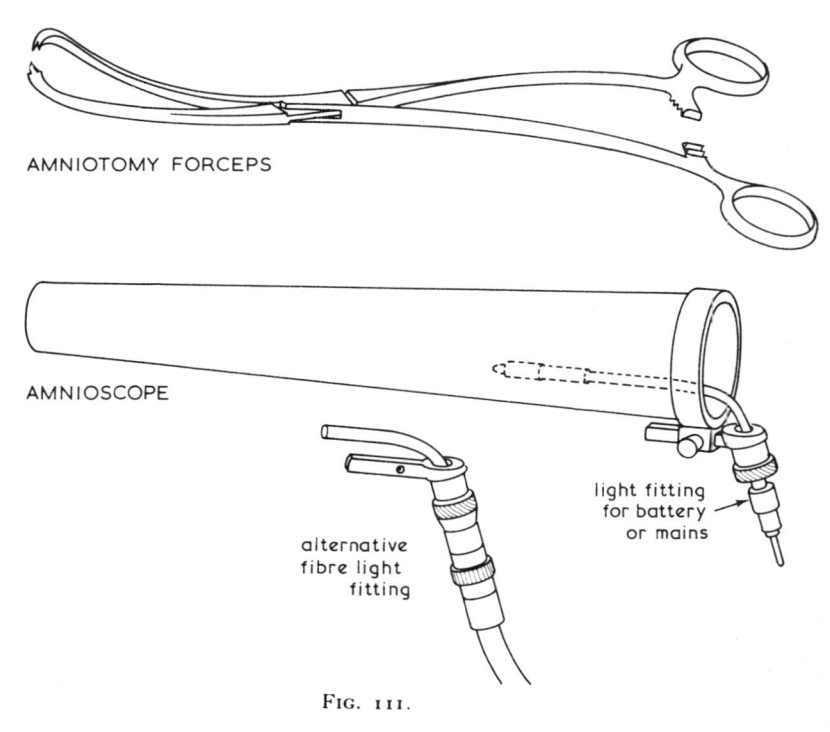

AMNIOTOMY FORCEPS

AMNIOSCOPE

alternative fibre light fitting

light fitting for battery or mains

FIG. 111.

INSTRUMENTAL DELIVERY

Obstetric forceps are used to hasten the birth of the baby, if the signs of fetal distress mentioned above are present, or if the mother is to be spared the exertion of the second stage, e.g. in heart disease. The two blades can be separated, so that they can be applied singly over the baby's head, locked together, and used to draw it out of the vagina. Forceps are not applied unless the cervix is fully dilated, and are only used on the head.

The patient lies in either the left lateral or lithotomy position, and the bladder should be empty. A general or local anæsthetic is necessary. The technique of extraction is not of importance to the nurse, whose most vital task is by regular and intelligent observation in the first stage to enable the doctor to hasten delivery in this way before maternal or fetal distress has become dangerous.

This is the traditional view of forceps delivery; it is used more readily now than formerly, because it is known that a short second stage is beneficial to the baby. The practitioner of active management does not favour a second stage lasting more than 30 to 45 minutes.

Another method of shortening the second stage is ventouse extraction. A cup is applied to the fetal head after the membranes have ruptured, and negative pressure is applied through it. Three sizes of cup are available, the one selected being that appropriate to the stage of cervical dilatation. Gentle traction can be applied during a contraction, and this encourages first cervical dilatation and then descent of the head. Ventouse extraction may be begun before the cervix is fully dilated, and takes up no space at the sides of the pelvis as do the blades of the obstetrical forceps. An œdematous lump or "chignon" is evident after delivery on the baby's head where the cup has been applied, but this soon disappears. Very occasionally the skin may be broken, and though this heals without trace, it is rather distressing for the mother, who must be assured that it is only transitory.

THIRD STAGE MANAGEMENT

Oxytocin and ergometrine injection BP (Syntometrine) is given when the anterior shoulder is born. The timing is important, or the placenta may be retained. Bleeding is minimal, and the third stage shortened to three to five minutes. By the time the midwife has coped with the baby, she is usually ready to deliver the placenta. One hand is placed on the fundus, and two fingers of the other are passed around the cord. Very gentle traction will assist the expulsion of the placenta.

CÆSAREAN SECTION

There are patients for whom delivery by the natural channels is impossible, or is dangerous to mother and child,

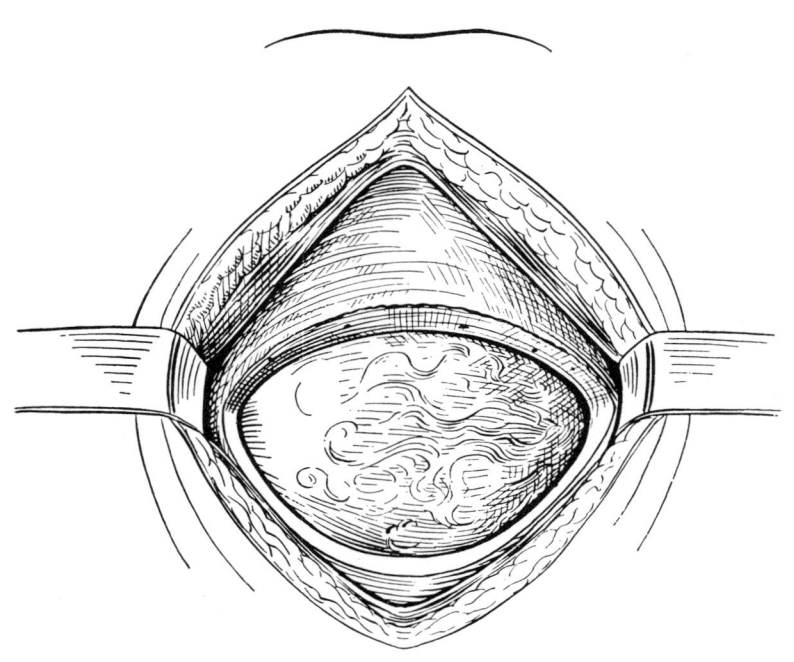

Fig. 112. Lower segment Cæsarean section. The abdomen has been opened and the uterus incised in its lower segment. The head is exposed and is the first part extracted.

and these patients are delivered by opening the uterus from the abdomen, and extracting the baby and placenta through the incision.

The patient is prepared in the same way as for any abdominal gynæcological operation, the uterus is exposed and a transverse incision made through the lower uterine segment. The baby is extracted and handed to the midwife, whose task is to see that respiration is established. Ergometrine is given intravenously, the placenta is removed and stitching up undertaken.

The baby, who has entered the world rather abruptly, is usually kept in his cradle for the first few hours, then the normal baby routine will be followed. The treatment of the mother combines the usual obstetrical attention, besides care of the abdominal wound, from which the stitches are removed on the eighth to the tenth day.

POST-PARTUM HÆMORRHAGE

Some blood is always lost during the third stage of labour and, if this loss exceeds 600 ml. (20 fl. oz.), it is termed a post-partum hæmorrhage. Such a figure is an artificial distinction since a patient who has lost blood before delivery or is anæmic may be severely affected by a quite moderate loss. Bleeding is less common if the active management of the third stage (described above) is practised.

The important fact is the effect of the blood loss on the patient; if she shows such signs as pallor, sweating and a rising pulse rate, medical treatment is indicated whatever the amount lost. Post-partum hæmorrhages can be sudden, large and alarming, and should the nurse be alone she must keep cool and treat her patient for shock in the way she has been taught until medical help arrives.

Bleeding may occur before the placenta is expelled and is then due to partial separation of the placenta. The uterine muscle cannot contract efficiently to constrict the bleeding vessels while the placenta is still present. Hæmorrhage will usually continue until the placenta is expelled but efforts to express it before it is completely detached will only increase the bleeding. Ergometrine, 0·5 mgm. given intramuscularly will cause the uterus to contract and will usually stop the bleeding. Ergometrine, 0·5 mgm, mixed with hyalase, and a combination of ergometrine and syntocinon 5 units both act more rapidly when given intramuscularly than ergometrine alone. If hæmorrhage is very severe, ergometrine, 0·5 mgm. or syntocinon, 5 units, should be given intravenously.

Hæmorrhage after delivery of the placenta is due to lack of muscle tone and ergometrine should be given at once. Massage of the fundus of the uterus through the abdominal wall will usually produce a contraction of the uterus that will control the bleeding.

If the placenta is retained in the uterus for more than an hour, it is usual to remove it manually under an anæsthetic and with full aseptic care as soon as the patient's general condition warrants it. Blood transfusions given promptly and in adequate quantities to patients who have suffered from post-partum hæmorrhage have saved many lives.

CHAPTER 15

CARE OF MOTHER AND BABY

THE PUERPERIUM

It is common for women to remain in hospital for eight to ten days after a normal delivery, though discharge after forty-eight hours to the care of the midwife and general practitioner is often possible and increasingly practised. During this time there are many important physiological and mental adjustments that the mother must make. She has to have a period of rest after the muscular efforts at labour; her pelvic muscles and ligaments which have been stretched during labour should recover their tone. The uterus must undergo the process of involution, by which its bulk decreases until it once again lies below the pelvic brim, and the raw placental site must heal. Lactation must be satisfactorily established, and she must learn to handle the baby and perform its toilet.

The chief points of importance in caring for her are these:—

(1) **Activity.** Immediately after delivery the mother needs rest and sleep, but from the second day onwards graded activity should help her regain her muscle tone, and avoid the dangers of venous thrombosis. On the second day she may begin breathing and foot exercises in bed, and this evening she may get up while the bed is made, and in many hospitals will be allowed her first bath or shower. Exercises and activity are gradually increased until by the tenth day she is capable of looking after her baby at home. The importance of post-natal pelvic floor exercises in the prevention of uterine prolapse is great.

(2) **Bladder Function.** Urinary retention, sometimes entire but generally partial, is not uncommon in maternity wards. Bedpans should be given regularly, and it is wise to measure the urine for the first forty-eight hours. The output should be high, as there is normally a good diuresis after delivery.

258 MODERN GYNÆCOLOGY FOR NURSES

(3) **Observation of the Uterus.** After delivery the uterus can be felt in the abdomen, with the fundus about 5 in. above the symphysis pubis. Its height should be measured each morning, and if involution is normal, it descends steadily until the tenth day when it is no longer palpable from the abdomen. Bladder and rectum should be empty when the measurement is made, and the patient lies flat on her back. The nurse locates the fundus with the left hand and steadies it, then measures the distance from the top of the uterus to the upper border of the symphysis pubis with a ruler.

(4) **Vulval Toilet.** After delivery a discharge of bright blood occurs from the vagina. This discharge, termed the LOCHIA, remains red for about three days, becomes brownish, and by the time the patient leaves, should be almost colourless. If the lochia remains red beyond the

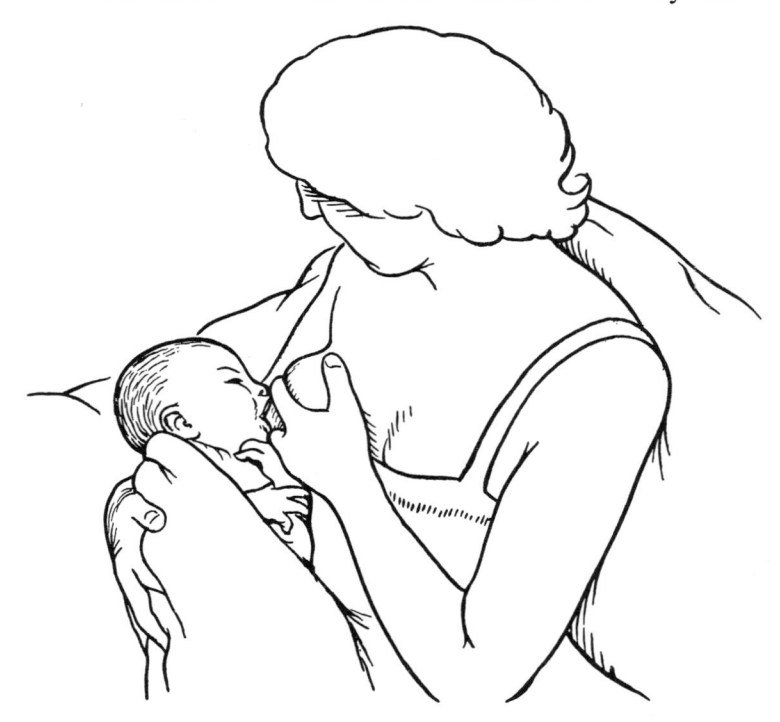

FIG. 113. Breast feeding. Notice that mother and baby are comfortably supported. The nipple is held between the tongue and hard palate, not between the lips, and the mother is depressing the nipple so that there is no obstruction to the baby's breathing.

expected time, or is offensive, infection or the retention of some shreds of membrane should be considered, especially if the fundus fails to descend at the usual rate, or there is any fever.

Vulval toilet is undertaken three times a day on the first day, then twice on the second day, after which the patient will usually be taking a daily bath. The nurse removes the pad with forceps, noting the character of the lochia, and places the patient on a clean bedpan. The vulva is irrigated with warm lotion poured from a jug, then thoroughly cleaned with wet swabs and dried. Stitches, if present, are treated as described on p. 129, and removed on the sixth day. A sterile pad is finally applied. Where the toilet accommodation permits the patient may be taught her own local toilet with sterile lotion and swabs after the first few days if no stitches are present. The nurse should then inspect the pads daily.

(5) **Breast Feeding.** The breasts are a pair of hemispherical organs lying over the anterior chest wall. At puberty, under the influence of hormones, they begin to enlarge from the deposit of fat within them. The secreting part of the breast consists of about twenty lobes of glandular tissue from each of which leads a duct. These ducts

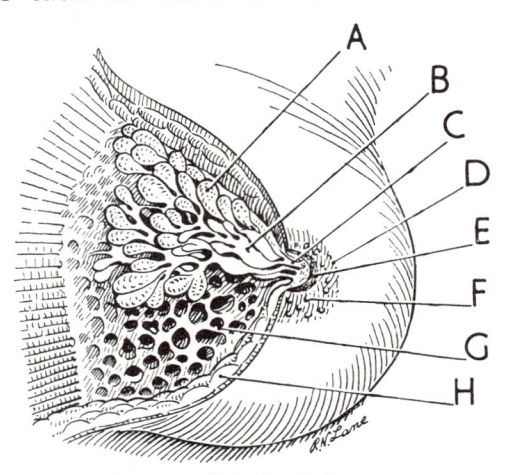

FIG. 114. The female breast.

A. Lobule.
B. Lactiferous sinus.
C. Lactiferous duct.
D. Areola.
E. Nipple.
F. Montgomery tubercle.
G. Connective tissue.
H. Fat.

converge at the nipple where they reach the surface. Within the nipple each duct dilates into a small reservoir for milk, the ampulla, and traction on the base of the nipple of the lactating breast produces a flow of milk. Surrounding the nipple is the pigmented areola on which open the ducts of Montgomery's tubercles from which a lubricant for the nipple is secreted.

The stimulus to lactation is the pituitary hormone, lactogen, but milk secretion will not continue unless the breast is emptied. The breasts begin to show signs of glandular activity soon after delivery but there is little secretion in a primigravida until the third day.

The main foodstuffs are present in the breast milk in the following proportions:

Protein   2%
Fat   4%
Carbohydrate   6%

The calorie value is 20 calories per fl. oz. (30 ml.).

The composition and temperature of breast milk are exactly suited to the baby's needs and the physical contact of mother and baby during breast feeding is a great satisfaction to both of them. The mother who wants to breast feed her baby is given every assistance by the nurse but the mother who has decided not to do this should not be made to feel guilty. Satisfactory formula feeds are available for artificial feeding.

On the first day the baby goes to the breast for a few minutes only at eight-hour intervals. This time is increased on the second day and, from the third day onwards, he is fed every four hours, gradually increasing the time until he is feeding for ten minutes on each side. Feeding routines are not rigid and allowances must be made for individuality but this is the usual pattern.

Before feeding the mother washes and dries her hands and nipples. The nipples are cleaned and dried when the baby has finished feeding. She should sit, well supported by pillows if in bed, or in a low chair. The baby lies in the bend of her arm and both mother and child should be comfortable and relaxed. The nipple must be held between the tongue and the hard palate and the baby's nose must not be buried in the breast or suckling will be interrupted because the baby must let go the nipple in order to breathe.

The baby must not be allowed to sleep at the breast with the nipple in his mouth lest sore nipples result, but he should be gently stimulated into wakefulness. Half-way through and at the end of the feed, the baby should be held upright and encouraged to bring up his wind.

If the nipples become sore, they may be treated after feeds with Friars Balsam, which is washed off with cetavlon before the next feed. The feeding should be supervised, and every effort made to prevent the nipples cracking, since this will mean taking the baby off the breast till they have healed, and expressing the milk until feeding is resumed.

(6) Diet. The fluid intake must be kept high to promote lactation and prevent urinary infection. The appetite is good, and the diet should be adequate to satisfy it. On the third day, in the normal case, an aperient like Senakot is given if necessary, and the bowels should be open daily.

(7) Rest. The mother's night sleep is somewhat shortened by the feeding routine, and all patients should be expected to sleep after lunch. Visitors should be restricted, especially during the first few days.

(8) Family planning. The woman who feels she has completed her family, or wants to postpone her next pregnancy, should be able to receive contraceptive advice if she desires it. Women who are breast feeding a baby, do not normally ovulate, and so cannot conceive, but if the pill is the contraceptive method used, this should be started three weeks before the baby is to be weaned. Those whose baby is bottlefed begin to take the pill three weeks after delivery.

BATHING THE NEWBORN BABY

The bath to be used should be disinfected with Deosan and detergent in hot water thoroughly applied with a mop, and then rinsed. The articles required are as follows:—

Bath of water at 38° C. (100° F.).
Soap and bath towel.
Sterile swabs, normal saline and olive oil.
Cord ligature, sterile scissors and collodion.
Receiver for used swabs.
Warm vest, gown and napkins. Safety pin. Blanket.
Rectal thermometer in vaseline.

Powder and baby cream or vaseline.
Baby's hair brush.
Scales and tape measure.

The nurse wears a mask, and perhaps a plastic apron under her gown. It will provide the nurse with valuable information about her technique if she takes the temperature at the beginning and again at the end of the bath; if it has fallen more than 0·5° C. (1° F.) she must improve her method.

The baby is weighed, and his length measured; this can be done most accurately by holding him up by the feet and measuring the distance from heel to vertex with the tape measure. The baby is wrapped in the towel and the nurse sits in front of the bath with the baby in her lap and washes her hands. With moist sterile swabs she gently cleans the lids and removes the cheesy vernix, which is the normal birth covering of the skin. Pushing swabs into the nostrils or ears is unnecessary and undesirable. The head is soaped with the hand, then the baby is held under the left arm with the hand supporting the neck so that the nurse can with the right hand rinse the soap from the head over the bath. He is returned to the lap and the head is dried. Opening the towel, the nurse with soaped hands rubs the front aspect of the baby and his limbs, looking at the same time for any physical abnormalities. She rolls him towards her, soaps his back and lifts him into the bath. The left wrist supports the shoulders and neck while the hand holds his upper arm; the right hand holds the ankles, and when he is in the water can be used to rinse off the soap. He is lifted out, put face downwards on the nurse's lap and his back is rapidly and gently dried. The creases may be lightly powdered, and a little cream or vaseline on the buttocks will facilitate cleaning. The napkin is laid over the buttocks and the vest over the shoulders if it is a front-opening one, and the baby blanket over all. The baby is lifted, the towel taken off the knees and the baby laid on his back. The vest is put on, the hands are rinsed and the cord inspected. If it has shrunk much another ligature should be applied and the cut surface painted with collodion. If a Hollister clamp has been used, the cord is left exposed and is cleaned daily with spirit. The clamp can be removed on the third day, and the cord will usually have separated by the sixth day. The temperature may be taken again, keeping the baby covered while it is registering, and taking this opportunity to see that the normal number of fingers and toes is present. The napkin is adjusted, and pinned with the left fingers inside it lest the baby is pricked. The gown is put on, the hair lightly brushed, and the baby is ready to go to the ward, where, if both are fit, his mother may hold him for a few minutes before he is laid on his side in his cradle.

The baby also has big adjustments to make as a separate individual. The contents of the intestine at birth are a dark green sticky material called MECONIUM and this must be regularly cleaned from the buttocks. Record should be kept of the passage of urine and meconium. The cord is not usually dressed, but is swabbed daily around the base with spirit until it dries and separates cleanly about the third or fourth day. The baby may be bathed daily, though some prefer not to do so until the cord has separated. By the ninth day the mother has been shown how to bath the baby, and subsequently does this herself under supervision until she goes home.

The baby's eyes need care, and it will be remembered that at birth the attendant cleaned the lids soon after the head was born. The instillation of a drop of silver nitrate 1% as a precaution against gonococcal ophthalmia has now been generally abandoned in this country. Any discharge from the eyes, however slight, must be reported at once, and if necessary a swab taken and specific treatment instituted. Unnecessary swabbing of the eyes should not form a regular part of the toilet.

By the tenth day it is to be hoped that the baby is feeding well, and has regained its birth weight, after the initial loss while lactation was being established.

ARTIFICIAL FEEDING

Breast feeding may be inadvisable because the mother has some condition like heart failure, or because the baby cannot suckle—perhaps because of prematurity, or for social reasons such as the impending adoption of the infant. There are also numbers of women who do not want to breast feed their babies. A suitable artificial feed must be found for the baby and the mother must be taught how to make it up and how to sterilize the apparatus at home.

Lactation can be suppressed by giving œstrogen. Stilbœstrol, 10 mgm., t.d.s., or ethinyl œstradiol, 0·5 mgm., t.d.s., is given for three days, then twice daily for three days, then once daily for three days, and a good supporting brassiere worn.

The basis of all artificial feeds is cows' milk, but this is not suitable for the newly born without modification. Cows' milk has twice as much fat and 30% less sugar than human milk and its protein is less easily digested.

Dried milks are the easiest kinds to store and the one advised is that with which the doctor has most experience. National Dried Milk is frequently used and the half-cream variety is roughly equivalent to human milk in its fat and protein content. It is low in carbohydrate but this can be remedied by adding sugar. The feed is made by mixing one measure of milk powder with 1 fl. oz. (30 ml.) of boiled water. A level teaspoon of sugar is added to every 3 oz. (90 ml.) of feed.

The baby should be introduced to the bottle by giving a little boiled water every eight hours in the first twelve hours, and then the milk feeds are started. The baby is offered an ounce (30 ml.) at first and this is increased on demand until at the end of a week 3–4 oz. (90–120 ml.) is being taken every four hours at each feed. If the baby is contented, its weight increasing and the stools normal, all is well. Most babies require about 3 oz. (90 ml.) per pound (0·5 kg.) body weight per day.

The bottles and teats must be cleaned and sterilized after use. Cleaning is done in soapy water with a bottle brush and the easiest sterilizing routine to teach the mother is the use of Milton: the clean bottle and teat are submerged in Milton, 1 : 80, for four hours.

The feed must be warmed to body temperature and the baby should be held in the lap as for breast feeding. Feeding should be done with attention, noticing the speed at which the feed is taken and keeping the bottle tilted so that the baby is never sucking air. If the hole in the teat is too small, the baby gets tired and gives up before it has taken enough, waking soon and crying for more. If it is too large, the feed is gulped so that wind and colic result.

Halfway through the feed, the baby is lifted to bring up his wind and, again, at the end. The napkin must usually be changed before he is laid down on his side to sleep.

SOME COMMON COMPLICATIONS AFFECTING THE BABY

There are many conditions that may threaten the baby during the neonatal period, and the more common of these are as follows:—

Congenital Abnormalities. Some congenital deformities are so severe that survival of the infant is not possible. Some, such as imperforate anus or œsphageal atresia, will be fatal unless surgically treated, and the nurse's observations in connection with feeding difficulties or failure to pass meconium are important. Some, such as extra digits, are trivial.

The causes of congenital deformities are not usually known. German measles in the first trimester of pregnancy can cause congenital deafness and cataract, and it is now known that some drugs taken in the same period can cause severe harm to the fetus.

Birth Injuries. During its passage through the pelvis, pressure may mould the baby's head until the parietal bones overlap. This is a normal phenomenon and the skull will soon return to normal. Sometimes an œdematous swelling (caput succedanum) appears over the vertex; this too will quickly resolve. A cephalhæmatoma is a subperiosteal hæmatoma, which can be differentiated from a caput because it is sharply bounded by the suture lines. It will disappear in a few weeks without treatment.

More serious are the intracranial injuries, which may threaten life or cause permanent mental harm. Babies who have suffered such injury are often limp and pale or ashen at birth, and breathing may be shallow or slow to start. Restlessness, twitching and a thin high cry are suggestive signs; vomiting and cyanosis in such a baby are danger signals.

The baby should be nursed in its cot, with as little disturbance as possible. The head-end of the cot is raised a little, and the air passages kept clear with a mucus extractor. Sedatives may be prescribed, and tube feeding may be necessary if after forty-eight hours the baby is not well enough to suck.

Jaundice. Breakdown of red blood cells occurs at a

brisk rate immediately after birth. If the liver is unable to deal adequately with the pigment produced, jaundice will result. A physiological form is common, usually starting about the third day and clearing within a week. No anxiety need be felt if the stools and urine are normal and the baby seems well. Jaundice occurring at or soon after birth and deepening, is of serious import, and may be due to hæmolytic disease of the new born (p. 208) or to congenital absence of the bile ducts. All jaundice should be brought to the notice of the doctor, and a record kept of the stools and urine.

Hæmorrhage. The clotting power of the infant's blood is low, and bleeding occasionally occurs from the bowel or elsewhere. It is treated by the injection of Vitamin K 0·5 or 1 mg.

Cold Syndrome. This condition is uncommon in hospital, and is due to loss of heat by the baby in cold surroundings. The child is limp, apathetic, and reluctant to feed. The temperature should be taken in the rectum by a low-register thermometer, and may have fallen to 28° C. (c. 82° F.). Warming must be very gradual, but once the diagnosis has been made, treatment is usually successful.

Infections. A scrupulous nursery routine is necessary to avoid infection of the baby, especially by staphylococci. Infections of the cord-stump, the skin, the conjunctiva, the respiratory tract, and the bowel may all occur, and stress is laid on their avoidance in all maternity units. The hands should be washed thoroughly after attention to a baby; all feeding utensils must be sterilized; baths must be clean; masks help to avoid respiratory infection; and nurses must not cuddle the baby against the cheek. This is the mother's prerogative.

THE PREMATURE BABY

The premature baby is one born before the gestation time is complete but, since this time is difficult to establish, the international definition is that the premature infant is one weighing 5½ lb. (2,500 gm.) or less at birth. On the whole, the weight is a fairly reliable guide to the chances of survival; a baby of less than 2 lb. (900 gm.) is not likely to live. A baby that would have been a big one if it had completed its allotted span in the uterus may, however, if born prematurely, weigh more than 5½ lb., but still require special care if it is to survive.

The causes of prematurity are fetal (such as congenital malformations), maternal (such as toxæmia, multiple pregnancy, injury, fevers) or unknown. The appearance of a baby of marked prematurity is characteristic. The skin is red, covered with downy hair (lanugo) and lacks subcutaneous fat. The head appears large for the body and the nails are short and soft. Inability to regulate the body temperature and muscular feebleness, that makes both feeding and respiration exhausting, are the main handicaps of the premature infant.

If it is known that a baby is being born early, preparations for its reception should be made. Since the body surface is large for the infant's size, heat is lost very easily and the surrounding temperature should be between 85 and 90° F. (30 and 32° C.). In an atmosphere as warm as this, dehydration will soon occur unless the humidity can be raised to 90%. These conditions can most easily be met in an incubator, but a small room which can be well warmed and where the air can be moistened by a steam kettle is satisfactory for all but the smallest babies. No clothes are necessary in an incubator and the baby is spared muscular effort by their omission. If nursed in a cot, he will need a gown with a hood to prevent heat loss from the body and head; a small fluffy napkin, and socks.

The needs of the baby may be considered under these headings:—

(1) *Maintenance of Respiration.* The air passages must usually be cleared at birth by a mucus catheter and attacks of cyanosis may require treatment by lowering the head of the cot, clearing the airway and, perhaps, by giving oxygen. High concentration of oxygen can cause blindness in babies by producing fibrous tissue in the eye behind the lens (retrolental fibroplasia). Therefore only low concentrations of oxygen are used and oxygen is not given for periods longer than the baby's need for it. Very gentle and regular turning of the child from one side to the other will help to prevent hypostatic pneumonia. The baby must not be allowed to lie on its back lest inhalation of vomit occur. Constant vigilance may be needed in the early days to keep the baby breathing.

(2) *Prevention of Infection.* Such a baby is very vulnerable to infection and a scrupulous barrier technique is used to protect him. No one with respiratory or skin infection should go near him; masks and gowns are worn, careful hand-washing is practised and feeds must be sterile.

(3) *Avoidance of Injury.* The baby is handled with extreme gentleness to avoid injury to skin or mucous membrane. Skin toilet is minimal except for the buttocks. Meticulous care is required both for feeding and in the use of the mucus catheter.

(4) *Suitable Feeding.* Feeding should not be started until the infant indicates by restlessness and sucking movements that it is hungry, usually two or three days after birth. Feeding the premature calls for skill, intelligence and devotion. Regurgitation of milk is a definite hazard to the airway and it is essential to find the right quantity, the right constituents and the most suitable means of giving the feed.

Glucose water is usually given at first, to avoid the dangers of a low blood sugar (hypoglycæmia) but, if expressed breast milk is available, it can be used diluted at first and then in full-strength. There are many suitable artificial feeds if breast milk cannot be obtained and the one chosen will depend on the pædiatrician's preferences. The amount needed at first is about 1 oz. (30 ml.) per lb. (450 g.) body weight per day and this is raised as the baby indicates a desire for more or becomes restless before the next feed is due. Feeds are not usually given at intervals of less than three hours as whatever method is used it is tiring for the baby.

A baby too feeble to suck is tube-fed. A catheter, size 4, is lubricated with glycerine and passed through the mouth into the stomach and, through this, the feed is introduced. It involves no exertion for the infant and is safe if the catheter is gently passed and the feed given very slowly.

A pipette was formerly recommended for weak infants but the danger of this is that the milk may be delivered faster than the baby can swallow it and fluid may enter the lungs. Whatever method of feeding is used, the head of the cot should be raised and the baby should be lifted into the upright position while wind is brought up.

(5) *Close Observation.* Constant assessment of the

CARE OF MOTHER AND BABY

baby's condition should be made. The temperature should be taken with a low-register thermometer; the passage of stools and urine should be recorded; the colour and breathing must be watched because, in frail babies, respiratory failure can occur suddenly; the baby's reactions and movements are an important guide to management.

(6) *Dietetic Supplements.* Extra vitamins are required and are most conveniently given in the feeds in a concentrated form such as Abidec. Iron will be required to correct the anæmia that commonly develops in premature infants. An injection of Vitamin K, 0·5 mgm., should be given to every premature baby at birth to prevent bleeding.

(7) *Handling.* Contact with its mother is the prerogative of every baby and a weak premature baby who spends a long time in an incubator is deprived of this. The mother often feels that she is able to do nothing for her baby and, indeed, usually goes home before the baby is able to leave hospital. This state of affairs should be remedied as soon as possible and a normal relation established between the two.

As the temperature rises to normal and the baby indicates, both by its appearance and movements, that it is recovering from its handicap, normal feeding and management may gradually be introduced.

POST-NATAL EXAMINATION

When the mother goes home with her new baby, she is going to a totally different situation from the one she left. In hospital she had no responsibilities or anxieties, and now she will have many. Breast feeding a baby is a great physical drain, and the nurse must try to picture the patient's difficulties on her return home and help her if possible to solve them. She can be assured that the health visitor will be calling soon, and will give her any advice she needs. An appointment should be arranged for a post-natal examination in a month's time.

This examination is a complete and thorough one, and may do much for the future health of mother and baby. She is asked about her progress since she left hospital, and if any troubles have arisen. She is weighed, the blood pressure taken, and the urine tested for albumin, these tests being of great importance if she suffered from toxæmia during pregnancy. A complete pelvic examination is made. First the perineum is inspected to see that the episiotomy or any tears have healed soundly. Then with a speculum, the cervix is examined for lacerations or cervicitis, and the character of any discharge noted and a cervical smear taken for cytological examination. Digital examination then determines the tone of the pelvic muscles, and ligaments, and bimanual palpation of the uterus will reveal if involution has occurred normally, and that no retroversion is present. The hæmoglobin is estimated, and she is given iron if any anæmia is present.

The patient is questioned on breast feeding, and whether the supply is adequate, and the breasts and nipples inspected. If lactation is not satisfactory she is given advice on how to improve it. The baby is weighed, and it is ascertained that his feeding routine and bowel action are satisfactory. The umbilicus, buttocks, eyes and skin should all be free from sepsis. If the patient's circumstances are suitable, she is recommended to take the baby regularly to the welfare clinic to check on his progress.

Careful examination at this stage may prevent much chronic ill-health later for the mother, and relieve her mind on some of the difficulties that always arise after leaving hospital. It is time well-spent in ensuring trouble-free progress for mother and baby.

LIFE AT HOME

The health visitor calls on all mothers after discharge from hospital, or when the midwife ceases attendance after a home delivery, to see if there is any need for special advice. Mothers of first babies often feel anxious when they assume sole responsibility for their baby; in hospital small problems about feeding and crying were solved by the staff, and these may assume major proportions when the mother is on her own. The health visitor is well qualified to give support and guidance on a wide range of topics, and to direct the mother to other agencies when necessary. Home helps, for instance, may in some circumstances be provided by the Social Service Department.

CONDITIONS COMPLICATING THE PUERPERIUM

The commonest complication of the lying-in period is

infection, and although the severe fulminating infections which, as "puerperal fever," caused so many deaths are now rarely seen, this is because of vigilance over their prevention, detection and treatment. Even minor sepsis must be energetically treated, for if it is due to an organism resistant to antibiotics it may become endemic in a maternity unit.

Puerperal infections should be seldom seen if a high standard of care is observed in the labour room and the lying-in ward. If they occur the bacteriologist may be able to help in locating the source of the infection and suggesting methods of eradication.

Puerperal pyrexia, which used to be defined as "any febrile condition occurring in a woman in whom a temperature of 100·4 °F. (38 °C.) or more has occurred within fourteen days after confinement or miscarriage." If a midwife is attending a patient in her own home she must obtain medical assistance if such a rise of temperature occurs, and the hospital nurse must inform the house officer. The patient and her baby should be isolated, and an examination made to determine the site of the infection that has caused the fever. It may be within the genital tract or outside it, so that a general as well as a local examination is made. Causes of pyrexia other than genital infections include the following:—

(a) **Mastitis.** Very marked pyrexia and general malaise may be caused by infection of the lactating breast. A tender reddened triangular area with its apex pointing towards the nipple is seen in the lower half of the breast. The part is engorged because milk cannot escape through the inflamed ducts, and an abscess will result if treatment is not promptly undertaken. If the baby is taken off the affected breast, the milk must be expressed either by hand or by pump to prevent congestion. Tetracycline or a similar antibiotic is given, and culture of the milk made to determine the sensitivity of the organism, which is usually a penicillin-resistant staphylococcus.

If inflammation persists and pus is formed, the abscess will be opened and drained. Aspiration of the pus and penicillin replacement is liked by some, but may prove rather a lengthy and inadequate method of treatment.

Mastitis may occur in an acute form early in the puerperium, but is commoner in the third or fourth weeks, after the patient has left hospital. A cracked nipple is a common site of entry for the infection, and patients should be instructed in the care of the nipples, and told the importance of seeking help if they become sore. Nurses working in obstetric units are often unaware of the incidence of breast abscess in their patients because this complication arises after they have left hospital.

(b) **Urinary Infection.** After delivery micturition is normal in the majority of women, but if the bladder has been bruised during a difficult forceps delivery, or if a low grade bladder infection was present before, cystitis may develop and even acute pyelitis. A mid-stream specimen of urine is sent for bacteriological examination, a high fluid intake is encouraged and treatment given on the lines indicated elsewhere.

(c) **Venous Thrombosis.** Clotting can occur in varicose or in normal veins in the leg, and an account of the symptoms and treatment will be found on p. 55.

(d) **Intercurrent Infection.** Fever may be due to some cause not directly connected with the delivery, such as influenza, tonsillitis or one of the acute specific fevers. Occasionally bronchopneumonia may occur if an anæsthetic has been given.

PUERPERAL SEPSIS

Genital sepsis is more important and more dangerous than the extragenital variety, and whenever the temperature rises during the puerperium the possibility of infection of the placental site must always be borne in mind.

Signs and Symptoms. Sepsis rarely becomes apparent before the second day after delivery, and is often much later. It may have been noted in the morning that the fundus of the uterus has failed to descend during the last twenty-four hours, and that the lochia are profuse, bright red and often offensive. The patient may complain of headache and malaise and towards evening the temperature begins to rise, and the pulse rate shows a proportionate increase. If the infection has spread upwards from sepsis in a perineal wound or in lacerations of the vagina she complains of burning pain locally and there is swelling of the perineum so that the stitches cause intense discomfort.

CARE OF MOTHER AND BABY

If unchecked, infection may spread in one or more of the following ways:—

(1) Direct spread. The uterus tubes and ovaries may become involved and local or general peritonitis may follow.

(2) Lymphatic spread is possible, as in all infections.

(3) Spread along cellular tissue occurs if cervical lacerations allow access to the parametrium by the infecting organism. Extensive pelvic cellulitis can result.

(4) Spread by the blood stream causes the most severe infections. Infected clots in veins may detach and cause abscesses in various parts of the body (pyæmia). The presence of organisms in the bloodstream (bacteriæmia) is common in many infections, but multiplication in the bloodstream (septicæmia) is only found in the most severe.

Methods of Infection. The organism responsible is often a streptococcus or staphylococcus; infections by *Ps. pyocyaneas* or *B. proteus* are less common, usually mild, but often difficult to eradicate. Gas gangrene is known, but is fortunately rare.

The organism may be one from the patient's own throat or skin, or may be one introduced by the medical or nursing attendants from their throats, hands or instruments. The bacteriologist is often able to trace the source of infection to the nose or throat of a member of the staff.

Predisposing Causes

(1) General factors. Anæmia, or toxæmia may have lowered the patient's resistance before labour; hæmorrhage is an important factor during labour.

(2) Local factors. Trauma; prolonged labour; instrumental delivery; cervical, vaginal or perineal tears; retained products of conception.

(3) Careless technique during vaginal examination or delivery.

Prevention of Puerperal Sepsis

While the decline in the maternal mortality of puerperal fever is due to the use of antibiotics, the declining incidence is due to an understanding of the modes of infection and better aseptic technique. Good antenatal care will reduce the number of women with septic foci such as infected teeth, and of long and difficult labours by preventing complications.

Treatment of Puerperal Sepsis

The cause of the infections must be sought as soon as fever is noticed. It may at once be evident, but if it is not, the breasts, legs, chest, pelvis and throat are examined, a mid-stream specimen of urine obtained and a cervical and throat swab taken. Penicillin injections are usually ordered at once, pending the bacteriologist's report, and anæmia is corrected by transfusion if necessary.

The patient and her baby are isolated in a well-ventilated room and if possible should have their own nurse. Fluids are given generously, and the diet, which usually needs to be light in nature, must contain plenty of protein. Scrupulous toilet is given to the vulva. In most cases response to treatment is rapid.

Even the most junior nurse working in a maternity ward must realize her responsibility with regard to the introduction and spread of infection. However excellent the routine of the ward, its effectiveness depends on the conscientious application by all the members of the nursing and medical team.

Pulmonary Embolism. This dreaded complication is less common than formerly, but the same need for vigilance in its prevention is necessary in the puerperium as is used for gynæcological patients.

Puerperal Insanity. Acute mental illness may arise in the puerperium, and the advice of the psychiatrist should be sought in connection with emotional disturbance. Sleeplessness is an especially important sign which the nurse must report. Acute mania may cause efforts at suicide or infanticide, and the patient must be allowed no opportunities for either pending her removal to a suitable hospital. Tragic cases are sometimes reported in the press, all the sadder because the prognosis for the patient is good if she and the baby are safeguarded in the acute stage.

INDEX

Abdomen, examination of, 27
Abdominal distension, post-operative, 49
Abdominal foundation set, 178
Abdominal operations, instruments for, 178
Abdominal pain, 10, 87
Abdominal wound, bursting of, 61
    infection, 60
Abortion, 228–36
    causes, 228
    complete, 231
    criminal, 229
    habitual, 232
    incomplete, 231
    inevitable, 230
    legalization, 228
    missed, 231
    septic, 232
    signs and symptoms, 229
    therapeutic methods, 232–34
    threatened, 224, 230
    tubal, 90
Abortion Act, 1
Abscess, tubo-ovarian, 84
Adhesions, 84, 86, 87, 89, 118, 160
Adolescence, 13
Adrenalectomy, 79
"Air hunger", 45
Airway obstruction, 41
Albuminuria, test for, 219
Amenorrhœa, 80, 96, 204
    causes, 96
    primary and secondary, 96, 98
    treatment, 98
Amniocentesis, 208, 209, 213
Amnioscopy, 213
Amniotomy, 252
Anæmia, 26, 30, 98, 104, 108
    in pregnancy, 217
Ante-partum hæmorrhage, 218, 224–26
Anterior colporrhaphy, 128
Anti-D globulin, 209
Aperient, 31, 49
Ascorbic acid, 31, 61
Asphyxia, 248
Aspirin, 47
Autosomes, 15
Avomine, 116, 214

Backache in pregnancy, 216
Bacteriological examination, 25
Bartholin's abscess, 148
Bartholin's cyst, 147
Bartholin's glands, 139, 151, 160
Bathing, newborn baby, 261

Bilirubin, 213
Biological incompatibility, 172
Biphasic reaction, 171
Birth injuries, 265
Bladder, catheterization, 31, 35, 51, 53, 120, 155
    drainage, 120, 150, 155
    function, 30
    infection, 39
Blood group, 30
Blood loss, 44
Blood pressure, 224
Blood transfusion, 30, 119, 136, 208, 256
    intrauterine, 209
Blood urea, 30
Bonney's blue, 34
Bottle feeding, 264
Brachial palsy, 23
Brain damage, 249
Breast, anatomy, 259
    carcinoma of, 79
Breast feeding, 259, 269, 270
Breast milk, 260
Breathing exercises, 30, 129
    pre-operative, 48
Broad ligament, 81
    hæmatoma, 90
Broncho-pneumonia, 48, 272

Cachexia, 70
Cæsarean section, 192, 254
Cancer. *See* Carcinoma
Cantor tube, 50
Carcinoma, 24, 29
    of breast, 79
    of cervix. *See under* Uterus
    of ovary, 69, 71, 115
        treatment, 72
    of uterus. *See* Uterus
    of vulva, 148
Carneous mole, 231
Catheter, 223
    indwelling, 40, 52, 128, 146
    self retaining, 38, 148
Catheterization, 31, 35–39, 51, 53, 120, 155
Cervical mucus, altering consistency of, 175
Cervical swab or smear, 26, 27, 112
Cervicitis, chronic, 153
Cervix. *See under* Uterus
Chancroid, 158
Chest, post-operative complications, 48
Chloretone, 116
Chlorpromazine, 121

INDEX

Chocolate cyst, 65, 72
Chorion epithelioma, 196, 236
Chorionic gonadotrophin, 10
Chorionic villi, 199, 200
Chromosomes, 15
  abnormalities, 213
Circadian rhythm, 6
Climacteric, 16, 18
Clitoris, 139
Codeine, 47
Coitus interruptus, 176
Cold syndrome, 266
Colostomy, 190–92
Colporrhaphy, anterior, 128
  posterior, 128
Condom or sheath method of contraception, 177
Condylomata lata, 163
Congenital abnormalities, 265
Consent for surgery, 28
Constipation in pregnancy, 216
Contraception, 1, 261
  methods, 172–77
Contraceptive pill, 80, 102, 166, 167, 176
Corpus luteum, 9, 10, 11, 89, 169, 201
  cyst, 65
  hormone, 80
Cows' milk, 264
Cryptomenorrhœa, imperforate hymen causing, 97
Culdoscopy, 194
Curettage of uterus, 99, 123, 180, 233
Cyclophosphamide, 77, 78
Cystitis, 51, 116
Cystocele, 126, 129
Cystoscopy, 117, 155
Cysts, Bartholin's, 147
  chocolate, 65, 72
  corpus luteum, 65
  dermoid, 68, 71
  follicular, 65
  malignant, 72
  ovarian, 64–69
    complications, 71
    operation for, 184
    treatment, 72
  papilliferous (papillomatous), 66
  pseudomucinous multilocular, 67
  rupture, 71
  serous, 66
  torsion, 71
Cytological examination, 26, 27, 112
Cytology, exfoliative, 112
Cytotoxic drugs, 77

Decidua of pregnancy, 201
Dermoid cysts, 68, 71
Diabetes mellitus, 143
Dialysis, 221
Diarrhœa, 116
Diathermy conisation, 153

Dienœstrol, 80
Diet, in pregnancy, 209
  post-natal, 261
Dilatation of cervix, 103, 123, 181, 202, 237
Dilatation of uterus, 180, 233
Döderlein's bacillus, 138
Dorsal position, 20, 114
Dramamine, 116
Dried milks, 264
Drugs, cytotoxic, 77
  for gynæcological operations, 178
  use in labour, 241
Dutch cap, 174
Dysmenorrhœa, 96, 100, 182
  primary or spasmodic, 101–3
  secondary or congestive, 103
Dyspareunia, 145

Eclampsia, 218–21
Ectopic gestation, 88
  ruptured, 90
  salpingectomy for, 182
Egg cell, 7
Endocrine system, 3, 5
Endometriomata, 65, 109
Endometritis, 83
Endometrium, 10
  three layers of, 12
Endoxan, 77
Enterocele, 126
Epidural analgesia, 244
Epimenorrhœa, 16, 96, 98, 103
Episiotomy, 156, 247, 248, 251
Ergometrine, 235, 253, 254, 255
Escherichia coli, 31, 217
Ethinyl œstradiol, 80
Examination of patient, 20–27
  bacteriological, 25
  cytological, 26
  equipment used, 24
  positions used, 20
  preparation, 24
  procedure, 26
  rectal, 20, 25
  trolley preparation, 25
  vaginal, 20, 25, 27
Eyes, care of, in newborn baby, 263

Fallopian tubes, 3, 11, 14, 63, 160, 198
  anatomy, 81
  cautery, 194
  diseases, 81–91
  infections, 83
  new growths, 88
  potency examination, 169
  pregnancy in, 88
  rupture, 90
  section through, 82
  tubal mole, 90
  tuberculosis of, 87

INDEX

Family planning, 172, 261
Fertility, 168–77
Fertilization, 14, 198
Fetus. *See under* Pregnancy
Fibroids of uterus, 104
  cervical, 106
  complications, 107
  degeneration, 107
  interstitial, 105
  signs and symptoms, 106
  submucous, 105
  subserous or subperitoneal, 106
  treatment, 107
Fibroma of ovary, 69
Fibromyomata. *See* Fibroids
Fistula, 155–57
  during childbirth, 156
  recto-vaginal, 156
  uretero-vaginal, 154
  urethro-vaginal, 154
  urinary, 154
  vaginal, 153
  vesico-vaginal, 154, 155
Fluid balance, 224
Foley catheter, 38, 129
Follicle-stimulating hormone, 7
Follicular cysts, 65
Follicular hormone, 79
Fothergill's operation, 128, 185

Genes, 15
Genital sepsis, 272
German measles, 265
Glottis, spasm of, 42
Glucose, 31
Glycogen, 138
Gonadotrophins, 7
Gonococcal ophthalmia, 166
Gonorrhœa, 1, 83, 152, 158, 159–61, 166
Graafian follicle, 7, 8, 10, 65, 169
Granulosa cells, 7, 9
Gumma, 164
Gynæcological operations, 178–94

Hæmatocolpos, 98
Hæmatoma, 60
Hæmodialysis, 221
Hæmoglobin, 30
Hæmorrhage, ante-partum, 218, 224–26
  in newborn baby, 266
  intraperitoneal, 88
  post-operative, 44
  post-partum, 255
  primary, 45
  reactionary, 45
  secondary, 46
Hæmorrhoids, 107, 215
Health visitor, 270
Heparin, 56, 58
Herpes genitalis, 165
Hexœstrol, 80

Hodge pessary, 134
Hollister clamp, 249, 250, 262
Home helps, 270
Hormones, 6, 7, 8, 9, 10, 195, 260
  corpus luteum, 80
  follicular, 79
  ovarian, 79
" Hot flushes ", 17, 19
Hot water bottles, precautions in use, 43
Human chorionic gonadotrophin
  (HCG), 195, 200
Hydatidiform mole, 234
Hydrosalpinx, 84, 86
Hymen, 139
  imperforate, 98
  causing cryptomenorrhœa, 97
Hyperemesis gravidarum, 216
Hypomenorrhœa, 96, 98
Hypothalamus, 6, 11–12
Hysterectomy, 29, 109, 115
  subtotal, 73
  total, 73, 109, 187, 236
    with bilateral salpingo-oöphorectomy, 73
  vaginal, 128, 136, 185
  Wertheim's, 43, 54, 74, 117–20, 188
Hysterotomy, 234

Ilium, 196
Incontinence of urine, 54. *See also* Stress incontinence
Indigo-carmine, 155
Infection, 60
  in newborn baby, 266
  intercurrent, 272
  precautions against, 25
Infertility, 107, 168
  and fibroids, 104
  investigation of, 181
Inherited characteristics, 15
Insanity, puerperal, 274
Insomnia in pregnancy, 216
Instruments for abdominal operations, 178
  for Cæsarean section, 192
  for dilatation and curettage of uterus, 180
  for Fothergill's operation, 185
  for ovarian cystectomy, 184
  for salpingectomy for ectopic gestation, 182
  for total hysterectomy, 187
  for vaginal hysterectomy, 185
  for vaginal operations, 180
  for Wertheim's hysterectomy, 188
Intercurrent infection, 272
Intertrigo, 143
Intestinal obstruction, 50
Intrauterine contraceptive devices, 175
Intravenous infusion, 44, 55, 119, 135–36
Ischium, 197

INDEX

Jaundice, 265

Kahn test and Price precipitation reaction, 164
Kidney function, 30
Kraurosis, 144

Labia majora, 139
Labia minora, 139
Labour, active management of, 251
  artificial rupture of membranes, 252
  epidural analgesia, 244
  first stage, 237
    analgesia, 241
  induction, 251
  instrumental delivery, 253
  mechanism, 247-50
  onset of, 237
  post-partum hæmorrhage, 255
  records to be kept, 242
  rupture of membranes, 247
  second stage, 242, 245
    analgesia, 244
  stages of, 237
  third stage, 250
    management, 253
  use of drugs, 241
  ventouse extraction, 253
Lactation, 6, 260, 270
  suppression, 264
Lactogen, 260
Langton Hewer's non-slip corrugated mattress, 22
Laparoscopy, 193-94
Laparotomy, 51, 187
Left lateral position, 20
Leucorrhœa, 151, 152
Leukæmia, 77
Leukoplakia, 143
Levator ani, 93
Ligaments of uterus, 94, 123, 187
Lignocaine, 215
Lithopædion, 88
Lithotomy position, 21, 114
Lochia, 258
Lung, massive or lobar collapse, 48
Luteinizing hormone, 7, 201
Lymphadenectomy, pelvic, 115
Lymphadenoma, 77

Mackenrodt's ligament, 94, 123
Malignant disease, 16
Manchester operation, 128
Manchester technique, 114
Mastitis, 271
Mayo-Ward operation, 128, 187
Mceonium, 263
Medicine, 2

Meigs' syndrome, 69
Menarche, 12
Mendelian dominant, 208
Menopausal menorrhagia, 16
Menopause, 5, 16, 18
Menorrhagia, 96, 98, 103, 106
Menstrual cycle, 173
Menstrual extraction, 232
Menstruation, 5, 10, 12
  changes in, 70
  disorders, 96
  onset of, 12
  pain during, 100
Mental illness, 274
Methotrexate, 236
Metropathia hæmorrhagica, 18, 99
Metrorrhagia, 96, 100
Microscope, 26
Micturition, 51, 53
  frequency of, 70, 106
  painful, 30, 85
Milk, cow's, 264
  dried, 264
  human, 260
Miller-Abbot tube, 50
Mittelschmerz, 10
Mons veneris, 139
Montgomery's tubercles, 204, 260
Morning sickness, 214
Morphine, 42, 46, 47, 48, 50, 58
Mother and baby, care of, 257-74
Müllerian ducts, 95
Myomectomy, 29, 108, 172

Newborn baby, artificial feeding, 263
  bathing, 261
  complications, 265-66
Nikethamide, 42, 58
Nipple, 260
  care of, 272
  secretion in pregnancy, 211
Nitrofurantoin, 52, 129, 150, 218
Nystatin, 141

Occlusive diaphragm, 174
Œdema in pregnancy, 215
Œstradiol, 79
Œstriol, 79
Œstrogen, 8, 11, 19, 79, 99, 102, 138, 142, 264
Œstrone, 79
Oligomenorrhœa, 96, 98
Oöphorectomy, 72, 79
Oöphoritis, 78
Ophthalmia neonatorum, 160
Ovarian cyst, treatment, 72
Ovarian cystectomy, 72
Ovarian hormone, 79
Ovariotomy, 72

INDEX

Ovary, 2
  anatomy, 63
  carcinoma, 69, 71, 115
    treatment, 72
  cysts, 64–69
    complications, 71
    operation for, 184
    treatment, 72
  diseases, 63–80
  fibroma, 69
  functional disorders, 78
  inflammation, 78
  removal, 72
  tumours, 64
  signs and symptoms, 70
Ovulation, 9, 10, 173
  determination of, 169
  suppression of, 176
Ovum, 7, 11, 14, 88–90, 169, 198
Oxygen, 44, 58
Oxytocin, 6, 234, 235, 251, 253

Pain, abdominal, 10, 87
  during menstruation, 100
  post-operative, 47
Papanicolau's test, 112
Papilliferous cyst, 66
Paracentesis abdominis, 75
  procedure, 76
  trolley preparation, 75
Paralytic ileus, 50
Parametritis, 130
Parentcraft classes, 211
Pelvic extenteration, 190
Pelvic floor, post-natal exercises, 257
  structure, 93
Pelvic lymphadenectomy, 115
Pelvis, anatomy, 196
  examination, 270
Penicillin, 160, 165, 232, 236
  gauze, 117
Pentothal, 42
Peristalsis, 15, 49, 50
Peritoneal dialysis, 221
Peritoneum, 3
Peritonitis, 50
Pessaries, discharge due to, 152
  medicated, 32, 34
  spermicidal, 174
  supportive, 133–35
  trichomonasidal, 140
Pethidine, 47, 129
Phenobarbitone, 219
Phlebothrombosis, 54
  post-operative, 23
Phthalyl sulphathiazole, 157
Pituitary gland, 6
  removal, 79
Placenta, 218, 224, 251
  expulsion, 253
  functions, 201
  removal, 255

Placenta prævia, 199, 225
Polymenorrhœa, 96
Population control, 1
Posterior colporrhaphy, 128
Post-operative care, 40–62
Post-partum hæmorrhage, 255
Pouch of Douglas, 93
  hernia, 126
Pregnancy, 10, 195–227
  activity, 211
  anæmia in, 217
  anatomy, 196
  antenatal care, 206, 213
  antenatal classes, 212
  backache in, 216
  breech presentation, 243
  clothes, 211
  complications, 207
    major, 216
    minor, 214
  constipation, 216
  decidua of, 201
  diet, 209
  extra-uterine, 88
  fetal circulation, 202
  fetal development, 202
  fetal monitoring, 213, 227
  financial grants, 212
  hæmorrhoids, 215
  insomnia, 216
  investigations, 207
  medical history, 206
  morning sickness, 214
  œdema, 215
  physical examination, 207
  physiology, 198
  post-natal care, 257
  post-natal examination, 269
  presentation, 212, 239, 242
    abnormalities, 243
  pyelitis, 217
  radiography, 207
  signs and symptoms, 203
  smoking during, 211
  special investigations, 220
  tests, 195, 201, 236
  toxæmia, 207, 218
  tubal, 89
  ultrasound investigations, 226–27
  varicose veins, 214
  vertex presentation, 239, 243
  weight control, 210
  weight increase, 218–19
  See also Labour
Prematurity, 266
Pre-operative treatment, 28–39
Procindentia, 126
Progesterone, 9, 11, 80, 99, 169, 201, 214
Prolactin, 7
Prolapse, 30, 51
  of uterus, 123
    operation for, 185

INDEX

Prolapse of uterus, post-operative nursing, 128
  of vagina, 123, 125
    post-operative nursing, 128
  operation for, 29
Prostaglandins, 234
Protein foods, 210
Pruritus vulvæ, 146, 215
Psychology, 2
Puberty, 12
Pubis, 197
Puerperal fever, 271
Puerperal infections, 271
Puerperal insanity, 274
Puerperal pyrexia, 271
Puerperal sepsis, 272–74
  methods of infection, 273
  predisposing causes, 273
  prevention, 273
  signs and symptoms, 272
  treatment, 274
Puerperium, 257
  complications, 270
Pulmonary embolism, 56, 60, 176, 274
  signs and symptoms, 57
Pulmonary infarct, 58
Pulmonary infections, post-operative, 48
Pulse, 45, 87
Pyelitis, 51
  of pregnancy, 217
Pyelonephritis, 51
Pyometra, 185
Pyosalpinx, 84, 86, 87
Pyrexia, 120
Pyridoxin, 116

Radiation burns, 156
Radiation sickness, 116
Radiography in pregnancy, 207
Radiotherapy, 77, 113–16
Rectocele, 126
Recto-vaginal fistula, 121, 156
Rectum, 3
Reproductive cycle, 6
  summary of, 10–12
Reproductive organs, 2
Reproductive system, physiology of, 5–19
Respiration, in premature baby, 267
  post-operative difficulty, 41
Retroversion of uterus, 131–35
Rhesus factor, 207–8
Rhesus negative, 208
Rhesus positive, 207–8
Rhesus typing, 30
Rhythm method of contraception, 173–74
Robert's sucker, 155
Ryle's tube, 43, 50, 87, 120

Salpingectomy, 90, 182
Salpingitis, 33, 83, 160, 161
  acute, 83, 84
  chronic, 83, 86, 103, 183
  tuberculous, 83, 87
Salpingo-oöphorectomy, 73, 86, 183
Salpingo-oöphoritis, 86
Scabies, 165
Senile vaginitis, 80
Serological tests, 164
Sex determination, 15
Sexual attitudes, 166
Sexually transmitted diseases, 158–67
Shaving, 32
Shock, 136
  after surgery, 31
  post-operative, 43
  surgical, 41, 74
Sims' position, 21
Skin, preparation for surgery, 31–32
Smear test, 26, 27, 112
Smoking during pregnancy, 211
Social counselling, 2
Southey's tubes, 75
Spasm of glottis, 42
Speculum, 27, 34
Spencer-Wells forceps, 250
Spermatogenesis, suppression of, 177
Spermatozoon, 15
Spermicidal agents, 174
Sporostacin, 141
Sterility, 168
Sterilization, 25, 28, 36, 194
Stilbœstrol, 80, 264
Stress incontinence of urine, 52, 127–28
Suction termination of pregnancy, 232
Sulphacetamide, 52, 218
Surgery, consent for, 28
Sweating, 41
Sympathetic denervation of uterus, 103
Syntocinon, 234, 251, 255
Syntometrine, 253
Syphilis, 158, 161–65
  acquired, 161
  congenital, 164
  early infectious, 161
  late, 163
  treatment, 165

Tampons, 13, 153, 174
Tetracycline, 271
Thiotepa, 77
Thoracotomy, 58
Thrombosis, 54
  prevention, 56
  venous, 272
Thrush, 140
Thrust, 165
Thyroid gland, 26
Thyrotoxicosis, 68
Tooney's needle, 245
Trendelenburg position, 22, 118

INDEX

Treponema pallidum immobilization (T.P.I.) test, 164
Trichomonas infection, 165
Trichomonas vaginitis, 139
Triethyl thiophosphamide, 77
Trocar and cannula, 75
Trolley preparation, for examination of patient, 25
   for paracentesis abdominis, 75
Trophoblast, 199
Tuberculosis of Fallopian tubes, 87
Tubo-ovarian abscess, 84
Tumours, pelvic, 27
Turner's syndrome, 15
Twins, 8

Ultrasound investigations in pregnancy, 226–227
Umbilical cord, 262
Uretero-vaginal fistula, 54, 154
Urethra, caruncle, 145
Urethritis, 51
   non-specific, 161
Urethrocele, 128
Urethro-vaginal fistula, 154
Urinary complications, 51
Urinary fistulæ, 154
Urinary infection, 30, 51, 218
   post-natal, 272
Urinary meatus, 38
Urinary system, 2, 53
Urinary tract infection, 51
   incontinence of, 54
Urine, retention, 3, 35, 51, 52, 53, 155, 257
   specimens, 36, 39, 117
   stress incontinence of, 52, 127–28
   sugar in, 143
   testing, 31
Uterus, 3
   anatomy, 92
   carcinoma, 18, 100, 109, 122
   cervix, carcinoma, 18, 30, 74, 100, 109, 110, 156
      cytology, 112
      diagnosis, 112
      nursing of advanced cases, 121
      signs and symptoms, 111
      treatment, 113
         radiotherapy, 113–16
         surgical, 117–20
      dilatation, 103, 123, 181, 202, 237
      erosion of, 152
   congenital abnormalities, 95
   curettage, 99, 123, 180, 233
   dilatation, 180, 233
   diseases, 92–136
   fibroids. *See* Fibroids
   inversion, 135–36
   ligaments, 94, 123, 187
   new growths, 104
      benign, 104

Uterus, new growths, malignant, 109
   physiology, 92
   post-natal observation, 258
   prolapse, 123
      operation for, 185
      post-operative nursing, 128
   removal, 83, 109
   retroversion, 131–35
   supports, 93
   sympathetic denervation, 103

Vagina, 3
   anatomy, 137
   congenital absence of, 95
   diseases, 137
   fistula, 153–55
   infections, 139
   new growths, 142
   painting, 34
   prolapse, 123, 125
   post-operative nursing, 128
Vaginal diaphragm, 174
Vaginal discharge, 22, 46, 85, 115, 121–23, 130, 135, 143, 151–53, 157, 159, 215, 258
Vaginal douche, 32, 46, 114
Vaginal fistulæ, 54
Vaginal foundation set, 180
Vaginal operations, instruments for, 180
Vaginitis, 135
   senile, 142, 152
   trichomonal, 139
Varicose veins, 107, 214
Vaso-motor symptoms, 17
Veins, varicose, 214
Venereal diseases, 158
Venereal infection, control of, 165
Venous thrombosis, 272
Ventouse extraction, 253
Vesico-vaginal fistula, 154, 155
Vesicular mole, 196, 234, 236
Virus oöphoritis, 78
Vitamin C, 31, 61
Vitamin K, 157, 266
Vomiting, carcinoma of cervix, 121
   chronic salpingitis, 86
   eclampsia, 220
   post-operative, 41, 42, 51
   pregnancy, 214, 216
   pyelitis of pregnancy, 217
   X-ray therapy, 116
Vulva, anatomy, 139
   boils, 142
   carcinoma, 148
   diseases, 142–51
   intertrigo, 143
   irrigation, 121
   kraurosis, 144
   leukoplakia, 143
   new growths, 148
   post-natal toilet, 258
   pruritus, 146, 215

Vulvectomy, 144, 148
Vulvitis, secondary, 143
Vulvo-vaginitis, 80, 139, 160

Warts, 165
Wassermann test, 163, 164

Wertheim's hysterectomy, 43, 54, 74, 117–20, 188
" White leg ", 56
Wound sepsis, 60

X chromosomes, 15
X-ray therapy, 72, 74, 115
XY chromosomes, 15